the MAGIC of
Massage

A NEW & HOLISTIC APPROACH

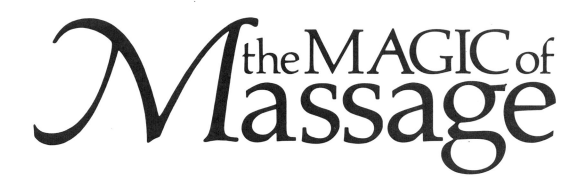
the MAGIC of Massage

by
Ouida West, M.Th.

Introduction by Dr Andrew Stanway, M.B., M.R.C.P.

CENTURY PUBLISHING
LONDON

First published in Great Britain in 1984
by Century Publishing Co. Ltd
Portland House, 12–13 Greek Street
London W1V 5LE

Reprinted 1985

Originally published in the United States in 1983
by Delilah Communications, Ltd.

ISBN: 0 7126 0314 X
ISBN: 0 7126 0316 6 (pb)

All photographs © 1983 by Una Fahy

All illustrations by Susan Margolis
(except pages 38, 39)

Book Design By: Una Fahy

Prints on page 11 supplied by
The Bettmann Archive

Printed in Great Britain by
Butler and Tanner Ltd.
Frome, Somerset

The recommendations in this book are not
intended to replace the advice of a physician.
Rather, they are meant to be considered for use
in conjunction with your physician's
recommendations.

Dedication

This book is dedicated to my parents, and the following people
for the profound influence they have had on my personal and professional life:
Stephanie Bennett; Louise Cardellina; T.C. Cherian, M.D.;
Rhoda Christopher; Una Fahy; Paula Fraser; Richard Gallen; Glenn Harz;
Sina Lee; Thomas Lemens; Michael Lobel;
Barbara Miesch; Diane Neault; Sandra Rosado; Gerald Paul Stone, Sc. Eng. D.;
Harold Wise, M.D.; and Sidney Zerinsky, M.Th., R.P.T., Ph.D.

Acknowledgments

Many thanks to the models who cooperated so patiently:
Cam Lorendo, Rochelle Sirota, John Burke, Madeleine Morel,
Paula Fraser, Lynette Mann, Jill Barber Petchesky, Rachel
Petchesky, Michael Macreading, Holly Wolf, Meg Wolf-Shapiro,
Jane Morgan, Jacqueline Carleton-Nathan, Steven Nathan,
Jennifer Paradine Carleton-Nathan, Suzie Brooks, Sabrina Brooks,
Dan Woldin, Louise Cardellina, Sharon Freedman and Noodge,
Wendy Spital, Tina Dudek, Antigone and Scott.

Thanks to the following people for their contributions:
Lanny Aldrich, Richard Schatzberg, Roger Mignon, Kathryn Greene, Amit Shah,
Maureen Charnis, Ed Caraeff, Nicholas Shrady, Antonio De Melo, Jerry Marshall
Virginia Rubel, Richard Amdur, Julianne Dobkin, Jo Irwin, Janice Johansen, Carolyn Barax

Special thanks to my editors:
To Jeannie Sakol for her brilliant insights, contributions and encouragement;
To Peter Skutches for his dedication in the early stages of the manuscript;
And to Melissa Smith, Paula Fraser, and Rhoda Christopher for their work.

I wish to express my great appreciation to T.C. Cherian, M.D.;
George Poll, D.C.; Alexander Teacher Jane Dorlester, C.S.W.;
Rhoda Christopher and Marjorie Conn, M.Th. & Ed.D., for helping to keep
my body and mind in good health throughout all the trials and
tribulations of writing and assembling this book.

Many thanks to those who were patient enough to
sacrifice many a massage in order for me to
complete this book.

Thanks to Glenn Harz for his support and encouragement, and
for providing me with a place in the sun to do the writing.

Extra special thanks to Una Fahy for her creative photography and design,
and to Susan Margolis for her beautiful and precise illustrations.

Finally, I wish to express my gratitude to Harold Wise, M.D.;
Sidney S. Zerinsky, M.Th., R.P.T. & Ph.D. and Mary Marks, D.C.
for reading and commenting upon my manuscript.

Table of Contents

Preface

My interest in the myriad functions of the human body began 12 years ago with the decline of my own health. I had begun to feel very ill and was unable to obtain satisfactory explanations or treatment. I quickly realized that I would have to take my health into my own hands and make the necessary life changes that would soon begin a reversal of the deterioration, or as it is commonly referred to, *dis-ease* that my body, mind and spirit was experiencing. After a great deal of reading, extensive research, and numerous courses and lectures, I finally felt prepared to begin to implement and experiment with what I had learned. Suddenly I noticed that my health was beginning to improve. My holistic approach towards achieving the vibrant health I now enjoy consists of a diet of only unrefined foods (80% raw and primarily vegetarian except for lean fish weekly), coupled with food combining practices and nutritional supplements, which the appropriate use of homoeopathic remedies compliment. Exercise, meditation, correct posture and movement as proffered by the Alexander Technique, Chiropractic adjustments and Massage Therapy in combination with the aforementioned dietary changes resulted in the alteration of my state of dis-ease to one of glowing, dynamic health.

With the return of my well-being I wanted very much to share my holistic approach with others, and my natural ability to touch seemed the most gratifying way to guide others to the realization of their potential for optimum health. Helping people to feel good about themselves makes it much easier for them to undertake the necessary changes to improve their overall health.

With the passing years I began to feel frustrated, in spite of the many victories over poor health that I had witnessed, because I could not help as many people as I wanted to. The opportunity to write this book has enabled me to present my approach to health to a greater number of people: a synthesis of the magic of massage and other methodologies that complement massage. While the material presented in this book is more than sufficient to start you well on your way to optimum health, there are many other recommendations that I would have liked to include, such as the regular consumption of high energy, vital foods like Bee pollen, Aloe vera gel, liquid chlorophyll, liquid acidophilis, brewers yeast, sea weed, wheat germ oil, pure garlic oil (undeodorized), and cod liver oil. Unfortunately, the reality of 192 pages made all of the additional suggestions impossible.

Self-help and helping friends and family are both beginning to be widely accepted. The many joys of being able to be personally involved in the betterment of our physical conditions, and the satisfaction experienced in successfully helping yourself and others, explains, I think the growing popularity of self-help programs. How wonderful it is to relieve someone's fatigue, headache, toothache, low back pain and more as well as replace their discomfort with energy and enthusiasm! Financial considerations as well as the realization that the responsibility for your health cannot be left exclusively in the hands of busy physicians and other health professionals has also contributed to the need for and the popularity of self-help methods.

Finally, although this book was written for the lay person, I feel that there is enough material to interest and be useful to the health professional as well. All of us, whether skilled in the art of massage, or new to it need to take our health into our own hands and experience the many benefits and pleasures discovered with a healthier approach to life and the magic of massage.

Introduction

Massage is probably the oldest healing art known to Man. It almost certainly started as a form of structured touching which people found produced positive results for their health and well being. Over the years almost every culture has 're-discovered' the magic of touch for itself and formulated its own system of massaging and touching for health.

Today, massage in its many forms is used to relieve stress, tension and emotional trauma; to heal physical damage to the muscles and skeletal supporting tissues; and simply as a pleasant thing to do as a form of communication within a relationship.

We in the UK are rather loath to touch one another —in fact, scientific research has found that we are at the bottom of the touching league of nations. How much then could we benefit from knowing and understanding more about various touching techniques? Obviously there are barriers to overcome in a reticent society such as ours, but once the joy or even the positive health benefits of massage have been experienced, there is no looking back.

But massage isn't simply a form of 'healthy behaviour.' It's a potent form of interpersonal communication. A couple who massage each other notice an almost immediate improvement in their interpersonal relationships. This comes about because the caring and loving required to perform a sensitive massage makes antagonism and anger less likely. The introduction of massage into an adult relationship can greatly enhance all communication within that relationship. As a result, the couple's sex life improves—often dramatically. In my experience of dealing with couples with marital and sexual problems there are few simple manoeuvres that are as effective as massage in getting them talking and eventually loving again.

Ouida West's book is unusual among massage books in that it treats the subject holistically and really gives the reader an understanding of what the subject means. She shows how the various types of massage differ and are related to one another, how massage can be used as a part of a healthy lifestyle to promote better health, and even how it can be a cure for certain simple conditions. On this latter point—just a word of caution. If ever you have a physical sign or symptom that doesn't get better fairly quickly using massage, don't delay seeking your doctor's advice. Massage isn't meant to be a cure-all, and to use it as such is to harbour unrealistic expectations.

Massage is here to stay in its many forms, from the most informal touching and cuddling of a hurt child to the highly sophisticated systems of acupressure and Shiatsu.

If Ouida West's book can break down at least some of the 'no-touch' barriers in our society and open a few doors to a healthier life it will have succeeded admirably in what it sets out to do. I am confident it will do just this.

Dr Andrew Stanway M.B., M.R.C.P.

CHAPTER I

What Is Massage?

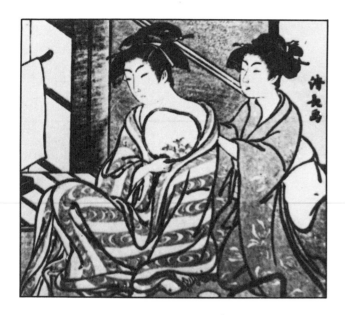 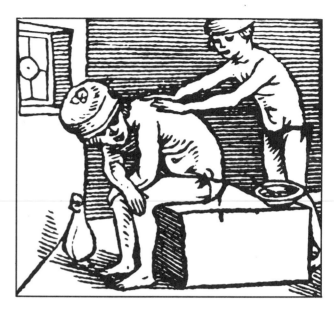

1) A BRIEF HISTORY OF EASTERN & WESTERN MASSAGE

The history of massage can be traced as far back as three thousand years before the birth of Christ. We can only speculate that humans prior to recorded history had an equally strong instinct to stroke or touch the body when it ailed, in order to console the afflicted, or speed up recovery. Even wild animals lick their wounds in an attempt to cleanse them and help them to heal. The following paragraphs briefly discuss all the major civilizations, beginning with the Chinese, that recognized and utilized the therapeutic benefits of massage.

The Chinese synthesized massage and gymnastics. Recorded history shows that the Orientals were using this form of massage at least three thousand years before the birth of Christ. A medical treatise known as the "Nei Ching," which is accredited to the Yellow Emperor Huang-Ti, contains the earliest Chinese references to massage. The Indian books of the Ayur Veda, written about 1800 B.C., refer to massage as rubbing and shampooing, which they recommend as a means of helping the body to heal itself. The medical literature of Egyptian, Persian and Japanese physicians makes many references to the benefits and usefulness of massage when attempting to cure or control numerous specific illnesses.

The Romans and Greeks, too, firmly believed in the benefits of massage. Homer, Herodotus, Hippocrates, Socrates and Plato, all among the greatest men of their times, all praised massage. Homer describes in *The Odyssey* the restorative powers for exhausted war heroes of rubdowns with oil. Herodotus states that massage can cure disease and preserve health, while Hippocrates, one of his pupils, believed that all physicians should be trained in massage. The writings of Plato and Socrates refer often to the use and excellent results of massage. Julius Caesar was pinched, i.e. massaged, everyday, because he suffered from neuralgia, and the famed Roman naturalist, Pliny, who was plagued by recurring asthma attacks, regularly received massage to help relieve these bouts. The Bible, too, contains innumerable references to the laying-on-of-hands as a method of healing the sick.

Massage continued to grow in popularity until the Middle Ages, at which time it lost its foothold in the medical profession because of a general atmosphere of contempt for the body and the physical world. Christianity placed an importance on the spiritual self that tended to exclude such earthly matters as the joy of physical well-being. All the sciences suffered great setbacks during this period of European history. Fortunately, the Renaissance brought back a renewed interest in the body and physical health. Much of the knowledge learned from the Eastern civilizations, as well as from the Greeks and Romans, was revived, and once again massage began to grow in popularity and develop as a science.

As the medical profession regained prestige, so too, did massage rise to new heights; for many prominent physicians incorporated massage into their approach towards curing the body and mind. Pare (1517-1590 A.D.) and Mercurialis (1530-1606 A.D.) were but two of the great physicians who integrated massage extensively into their medical practices. Ambroise Pare's methods proved to be so successful that he became the physician to four of France's kings. Mercurialis, a widely acclaimed Italian doctor, wrote a well-received treatise on massage and gymnastics that won him great fame and a rank among Italy's most prestigious physicians. The attending physician to Mary Queen of Scots led her to health in 1566 with his use of massage. Her condition was considered very grave and recovery was expected to be quite lengthy, but the doctor hastened her improvement through the application of massage techniques.

Massage took another great leap forward with the work of Per Henrik Ling. Ling, a native of Sweden, traveled to China and brought back some remarkably effective techniques of massage which he then assembled into a system known as "The Swedish Movement Treatment" or "The Ling System." There were many other physicians prior to and after Ling who contributed to the wealth of information now available on massage. Although they are too many to mention here in this brief history of massage, the bibliography lists numerous reference books which provide some

background in the history of massage. *Massage, Manipulation and Traction* by Sidney Licht, M.D., published by Robert E. Krieger Publishing Company, is one of the more detailed sources.

Currently, Swedish Massage and Japanese Shiatsu are the most popular methods of treating the body in Europe and on the North American continent. Shiatsu has recently been gaining a following of significance among practitioners and lay people. Even the medical profession is now beginning to take note of this intricate system of meridians and pressure points. There are many systems, some of which arose independently, currently in use in Europe and in North America, but the majority of them are off-shoots of either Swedish or Shiatsu. Some of the more popular independent and spin-off systems include: Rolfing, Soma Massage, Chiropractic, Touch For Health, Reflexology, Acupressure, Alexander Technique, Feldenkrais Method, Polarity and Barefoot Shiatsu.

2) THE MAGIC OF MASSAGE IS A GIFT

Massage seems magical because of the lack of scientific data explaining the body's complex systems, especially the meridian system. The magic lies, too, in the doer's ability to channel those mysterious life forces, that, when allowed to flow through us, make whatever we do more powerful and indeed quite magical. The Japanese speak of the hara as the place within the body where the essential energy of that body resides. It is in your hara, one-and-a-half inches below the navel, that you can find the magical strength to do what you are usually unable to accomplish. Don't be disturbed by the word *hara,* and don't worry if your knowledge of eastern philosophy is not comprehensive. Translated into lay terms, let your instincts be your guide. When you function on a purely instinctual basis, you are automatically in touch with those magical forces that allow you to sense things which normally escape your awareness. Instinct will usually, if heeded, guide you through many situations easily, gracefully and harmlessly. Apply the magic of those instincts to massage, and you will be able to sense where to touch, how to touch, and for how long in order to make your receivers feel better and even heal themselves.

The ability to give a magical massage without training or experience is a gift. Some people seem to be born with it. Most people, however, must learn how to give a magical massage. It may be learned more easily when one is desirous of mastering the art, and wishes to help someone feel better. Put your ego aside and listen to what the receiver's body is telling you. Let your instincts guide your hands as you fill your being with love and allow your compassion to flow from you to the receiver. If you are a clumsy person, do not despair. Massage from your hara, your center, and you too will be able to give a magical massage.

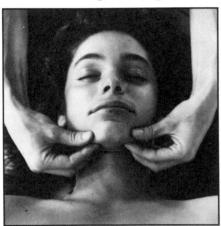

Massage is also a gift because you are giving your time to someone. You could just as easily choose to pursue a favorite pastime like playing tennis or watching television. Instead, you have chosen to spend a certain amount of your time giving of yourself to someone special or someone in need.

Massage is a gift in another way too. You, as the doer, are offering your receiver the gift of both physical and psychological health. It is a known fact that massage improves circulation of the blood and lymph, and that most conditions will improve if the circulation of these two vital fluids is encouraged. Therefore, while you are massaging your partner or friend, be fully aware of the benefits you are providing as you work.

Most of us do not get touched enough. Even though you may have an active sexual life, that does not mean you are receiving enough non-sexual touch. Experiencing massage by loving hands can help adults and children fulfill their needs for touch. Exchanging complete massages once a week or giving a quickie massage when it is needed helps to keep you feeling healthy and happy, as well as in touch with yourself and other human beings.

Finally, the ability to receive a massage is a gift, and many of us simply don't know how to accept a gift. It is often easier to give than to receive. The ability to let go and allow the doer to penetrate into your essential being to make you feel better must sometimes be learned. Not only is it the responsibility of the doer to make the massage successful, but also you, as the receiver, must help to make it work by allowing the doer to give.

The magic of massage is a gift in every sense of the word. If you are not one of the more fortunate people born with this gift, extend yourself and learn its magic so that massage can become an integral part of your life.

3) THE PSYCHOLOGY OF MASSAGE

Your state of mind when giving a massage is of utmost importance. Unless your feelings, awareness and motivation are unusually pure in nature, you will transmit your tensions to the receiver. If your tension levels are extremely high, chances are that your receiver will find the massage insensitive, indifferent or perhaps hostile. All life is composed of atoms. Atoms vibrate. The excitability of atoms is a known scientific fact, so watch your vibrations. If they are too rapid because of emotional upsets, either calm yourself or schedule the massage for another day.

If you are sick or feel like you might possibly be coming down with a cold or flu, do not give a massage. One obvious reason is that you may infect the receiver. Apart from that you must also realize that your energy level will be depleted. Not only will you run the risk of making yourself sicker, but also you will probably not be able to give a satisfying massage.

The most important rule to remember when giving a massage is to let your instincts be your guide. If you suddenly feel that you should touch a particular part of the body in a particular way, don't hesitate. Make a smooth transition from the technique you are presently implementing to that part of the receiver's body which is calling you, and employ the stroke or apply the pressure that is required to satisfy your instincts. Do not allow your ego to interfere while giving a massage because it will result in a less sensitive approach. Focus your mind on the receiver's tensions and fears, and watch them dissolve. Focus, coupled with your instincts, will enable you to feel the tension and fear hidden deep within the joints, muscles, organs and bones of the receiver. Imagine that you are a detective. Locate the assailant hiding in a joint, muscle, organ or bone, and dispose of the culprit.

It is not always easy to rid the body of its stored tension and/or fear. Once you locate a villain, try to coax it out by using the appropriate stroke or application of pressure. If you do not succeed after a reasonable amount of time, abandon your efforts for a while. Return to the area later, several times in one massage if necessary.

Humans tend to guard their tensions and fears as if they were precious jewels. Do not be overly aggressive when trying to dissipate them. Unwanted as these aspects of their psyche may be, most people are nevertheless reluctant to abandon any part of themselves. Allow love and compassion to come through your touch to show the receiver how much better the body will feel.

Many people attempt to bury tensions and fears within their bodies with the hope that the fears will remain a secret from themselves and the world. Though tensions may stay hidden for a while, they will eventually return in the form of bodily aches and pains. By this time the sufferer has no idea what the real problem is. A clever doer or massage therapist can communicate with these tensions and by compassionate manipulation can dissolve them. The doer may find it necessary to address the affected areas many times before the tensions disappear. One aid in this process is praise. As you massage an affected area, utter words that will encourage the receiver to let go and to feel good. If you sense the slightest release, offer a compliment like, "That was good! Now let's try for a little more." If the receiver releases all or a great deal of the tension and fear, exclaim, "Oh that was beautiful! You really let that go!" We all like to hear we're beautiful.

Many people have little idea where or to what degree they are holding their tension. Often they may believe they are relaxed, but you are confronted with rigid limbs. Don't criticize or try to force the receiver to admit to a tension the receiver may not be ready to accept. It's best to say, "Oh, I think I've found some tension here. Let's see if we can work together to let it go." Often the person will relax further if you are encouraging, because the receiver will no longer feel threatened or alone in the struggle. When the receiver does release, don't forget the compliment.

The use of imagery is helpful in encouraging some people to release stored tensions and fears. Perhaps the image of a rag doll to suggest that they relax their limbs, or ask them to think about something that makes them feel happy and peaceful, like a ship at sea. You can even be sneaky, if you know the receiver well enough. Casually mention something you know makes the receiver feel good to drive away whatever worries that may presently preoccupy the receiver's mind.

Most people hide their misery in the same spots, most commonly in the neck, shoulders or lower back. Repeated recognition of these storage areas will help to discourage further build-ups and will thereby encourage a less tense and freer body and mind. One last caution to the doer, do not allow the negativism that is leaving the receiver's body to fill yours. As the tension is released, neutralize it and send it away from your finger tips into the atmosphere. Better yet, try to dissipate it outward even before it reaches your fingers. One method of neutralizing negative energy as it leaves the receiver's body is to visualize its transformation into something positive like a bouquet of wild flowers or a ray of sunlight or a fish swimming happily away.

CHAPTER II

Why Massage?

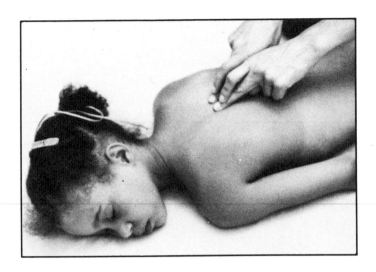

1) GENERAL REASONS TO MASSAGE

To massage or touch with the intention of relieving pain is an instinct basic to human nature. Since primitive times humans have touched and massaged themselves or others as the need has arisen. There are many instances, however, when it is more effective to touch a part of the body distant from the location of the pain. Our knowledge of distant-point therapy has been learned mostly through trial and error. Someone with a toothache, perhaps, accidentally hit the inner upper edge of the humerus bone on the same side as the aching tooth, and voila! The toothache disappeared. Likewise, someone with a headache may have received a blow to the outside of the thigh, midway between the hip and the knee, and the headache vanished. Discoveries like these were probably passed on by word of mouth from generation to generation. Eventually, though, they were recorded, and complex systems establishing the relationships between seemingly unrelated areas of the body evolved. The Chinese Acupuncture Meridian System and related disciplines which utilize distant-point therapy are discussed in Chapter III, Section 5 of this book.

When many Westerners think of massage, they think of health clubs or spas and a vigorous process of kneading, rubbing, pressing and slapping. Massage, however, can also be quiet, slow, penetrating and gentle. I define massage as any touch that is capable of evoking a change in the body. Even the lightest touch, when properly executed, may effectively stimulate circulation or alter the flow of energy within the body. Gentleness, as well as firm, penetrating pressure and a subtle, feathering motion, must also be considered valid massage techniques, for these methods have proven useful in relieving specific types of tension or pain. Massage, then, as the term is used in this book, refers to any type of touch.

Occasional massage treatments have been known to effect dramatic changes in both body and mind. However, to relieve or cure most physical and emotional problems, regular massage sessions are generally necessary. Based on my definition of massage as touch, I would like now to describe what massage, on a regular basis, can accomplish for your body and mind.

- Deep relaxation is induced by massage

- The release of tension in regular massage sessions often enables the receiver to overcome long-standing emotional turmoil because renewed energy becomes available to aid in coping with them

- Greater achievements are possible with renewed energy and a cleared mind

- Self-esteem improves

- The body and mind can be stimulated without the negative side-effects of caffeine or drugs

- Mental and physical fatigue is relieved

- Chronic neck and shoulder tension can be released

- Muscles receive an increased blood supply of nutrients that help to improve their functioning

- Calf cramps and other muscle spasms can be eliminated

- Waste products that accumulate in muscles after vigorous exercise can be removed to prevent soreness and aching

- Muscle tone can be improved, and muscular atrophy, due to forced inactivity, can be reduced

- Massage is a form of passive exercise that can partially compensate for lack of exercise

- Chest pains related to tight pectoralis muscles can be eliminated and a tension-causing fear of heart attack alleviated

- Fat stored in your tissues may be reduced

- Massage dilates blood vessels to improve circulation

- Arthritis patients experience relief because improved circulation to the joints reduces inflammation and pain

- Directly massaging the hands helps to relieve and sometimes eliminates neuralgic, arthritic and rheumatic disorders

- Bursitis responds favorably to massage

- Sprains heal more readily

- Fractures, breaks and dislocations take less time to heal

- Adhesions can be prevented or broken down to effect greater mobility

- The function of every internal organ can be improved, directly or indirectly, by the application of the many different techniques

- Digestion, assimilation and elimination can be improved

- The detoxifying function of the kidneys is increased

- Massage heightens tissue metabolism

- The lymphatic system is flushed by mechanically eliminating toxins and waste

- Massage returns blood to the heart thereby assisting in cardiac functions

- Massage can benefit anemics by increasing the number of red blood cells

- Eyesight and hearing can be improved

- Nasal congestion and sinus conditions improve dramatically and often totally disappear

- Sore throats can be encouraged to heal more quickly. If a sore throat is treated within the first hour, it can often be averted

- All types of headaches (Gall Bladder, Liver, Stomach, Large Intestine, emotional and migraine) can be eliminated

- The balding process can be stopped, reduced or reversed through frequent massaging of the shoulders, neck and head, and by making contact with the neuro-vascular holding points

- Wrinkles can be lessened due to improved circulation

- Back pain can be relieved

- Body fluid in the legs and arms can be reduced to decrease swelling and provide relief to tired or aching limbs

- Tired, burning, stinging or aching feet can be rejuvenated

✿✿✿✿✿✿✿✿✿✿✿✿✿✿✿✿

Massage is essential to your total good health. Unfortunately, most people consider massage a luxury. I disagree entirely, for everyone, regardless of age, will benefit from regular massage sessions. Given the daily pressures of the modern age, massage is a necessity. If you cannot massage yourself or exchange massages with a partner or friend, I recommend massage on a regular basis with a trained practitioner. If money is a problem, consider bartering services for massage sessions. Perhaps you could teach, baby-sit, or do light housekeeping in return for professional treatment. If you really want a massage, you can find a way to get it.

In any case, a basic understanding of massage is advantageous, because you will be able to help others or yourself when you least expect it and when it's needed most. One day when I was eating lunch in a restaurant, I heard a muffled scream from the kitchen. I peeked into the kitchen to see what had happened, and discovered the chef had cut her index finger. It was bleeding profusely. She bandaged it and managed to stop most of the bleeding, but the finger was throbbing. She found it difficult to continue working, and no one was there to relieve her. I asked if she would like me to stop the pain. She asked if I had an aspirin. "No," I said, "but I do know an acupuncture pressure point that will relieve the pain." Although she looked skeptical, she was desperate. I pressed firmly into her cheekbone, alongside the flare of her nose, for 60 seconds. When I released my pressure, the pain had stopped. She was startled, and looked at me as if I were a magician. I explained that the meridian or energy pathway for the large intestine begins near the base of the index fingernail, travels up the arm and over the shoulder, then up the neck onto the face, where it terminates next to the ala of the nose.

(See Meridian Illustration # 3 on page 39.) It is possible to relieve pain that occurs at one end of the meridian by applying pressure at the other end. I instructed her to press the same terminal point, should the pain recur. When I returned to the restaurant several weeks later, the chef told me that her finger had begun to hurt a few hours after I had held the pressure point. She had then held the point herself for about one minute, and the pain had never again returned. She also mentioned that the finger had healed more quickly than usual. Evidently she cut her finger often, so she had many instances for comparison.

Another incident that proved acupuncture pressure points a valuable first-aid treatment occurred when I was walking on a beach one summer day. I witnessed a young guy punch another in the nose and walk away. The victim was lying on the sand and looking rather stunned when I reached him. I asked if he would like me to stop the pain and reduce the swelling of his left eye. "Why not," he muttered. I took the toe next to the big one and squeezed it for several minutes. In a few seconds the pain in his eye had begun to subside. At the end of three minutes the swelling had begun to go down. I instructed the fellow to squeeze the toe frequently for the next few days in order to help his eye to heal. I also suggested that he get some ice at the beach snack bar and apply it immediately to the swelling. He was too stunned to ask why pressure to the toe had alleviated the pain in his eye. It had worked because the stomach meridian begins under the eyes, travels down the face, neck, trunk and legs, and terminates near the nail of the second toe. (See (Meridian Illustration #1 on page 38.) Again, the meridian principle applies. If injury to the body occurs at a point near the beginning or end of a meridian, it can be treated by applying pressure to the acupuncture pressure point farthest from it on that meridian. (See the Meridian Chart on pages 38 and 39 for further possibilities.)

Massage seems a lot like magic, because you see something happen, but you don't quite understand why. Don't worry about not understanding why. Scientists will, no doubt, eventually be able to explain why acupuncture, acupuncture holding/

pressure points and allied practices are so remarkably effective. Until then, use the techniques and reap the benefits. Not only can massage greatly improve your physical and emotional well-being, but it also may enable you to help yourself and others cope with everyday tensions, many ailments and the unexpected injury.

2) WHY MASSAGE FOR COUPLES?

Chapter IV, How To Give A Complete 60-Minute Body Massage, is geared to partners or friends who want to give each other a thorough massage once a week. Partners who exchange massage on a regular basis inevitably develop a deeper, more meaningful relationship. As trust, understanding and communication improve, your partner becomes your friend as well as your lover.

Too many relationships are based primarily on sex. There comes a time, usually after a year, when the sexual passion in most relationships becomes less intense, less frequent and sometimes less satisfying. At this point many relationships go into a decline. Both parties begin to feel that they are no longer as sexually attractive or attracted to each other as they were before. Insecurities and rejection set in, and partners soon discover they can no longer communicate on any level. Relationships that are failing can usually be revived through regular massage because massage helps partners to put their problems, their emotional needs, their sexual desires, themselves and each other into proper perspective.

Massage can improve and heighten the sexual experience. For those who feel they already have a good sex life, massaging for ten to twenty minutes before sexual activity can heighten an already satisfying experience. Massage enhances sex with sensuality. The ability to be sensual can be learned, or re-learned. By massaging the non-sexual parts of the body, partners can express the depth of their feelings in a purely sensual fashion. Oils may be used to further enhance the pleasurable physical sensations of mutual stroking, feathering and kneading. The neuro-vascular holding

points for the sexual organs can also be wonderfully stimulating. Massage techniques can make a sex life fuller and more rewarding by bringing partners closer together before actual sexual gestures are made. Original techniques can be created too. Indeed, they will often evolve naturally, evoking equally free and natural responses.

Massage helps to release tension, re-establish communication and effect a flow of uninhibited expression between partners in a relationship, even after long periods of withdrawal and strain. Any number of circumstances can strain a relationship, and a tension headache is one of the most common. It takes only a few minutes, however, to release the blockages causing the headache. There are points that, when held, release anxiety and thus make it easier for a partner to cope with an emotionally charged situation and physical or psychological trauma. Repeated use of these points will help the partner to overcome shock more quickly and with less pain than usual, and will reduce the amount of tension found in the relationship.

A quickie massage, exchanged after a long hard day in the office or home, enables partners to enjoy the evening together. It frees them from the tensions of working in an office or looking after a family that can often become overpowering. Too many couples spend nights quarreling or complaining about how exhausted they feel. After the fifteen to twenty-five minutes it takes to exchange a quickie massage, they would feel refreshed and could enjoy an evening at home, go out to dinner, see a movie or visit a friend.

Massage can also be extremely useful during times of illness. When disease strikes a member of a couple, the other is often plagued by feelings of helplessness. The thought that there is nothing you can do to improve your loved one's condition is apt to make you sick and your partner sicker. Most illnesses can be improved, controlled or cured through the use of the correct pressure points and other massage techniques. Furthermore, if you and your partner massage each other while you are both still healthy, you will avert many unnecessary illnesses. The inclusion of regular massage exchanges in your weekly agenda will reward you, not only with fewer aches and pains, but also with more energy and enthusiasm. The two of you together will enjoy a generally improved state of health in body and in mind.

In short, massage is one of the nicest ways of saying "I Love You." No words need be spoken, for the offer of a massage, when your partner is feeling low or exhausted, says it all. It is a special kind of gift, a unique expression of yourself, your compassion and your love.

3) WHY MASSAGE YOUR CHILD?

Massage strengthens and solidifies the parent-child bond. Parents should begin massaging their child while it is still in the womb. All too often

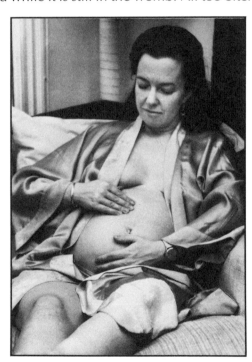

mothers have little physical contact with their child prior to delivery. Most mothers can locate the child's head at different times during the pregnancy and can determine whether the child is sleeping or awake, but too few of them spend enough time lightly touching and massaging the growing fetus through the abdominal wall. Massage helps the mother to understand and experience the child subliminally before it is born.

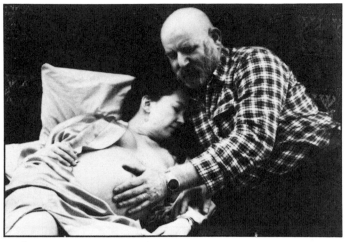

Fathers should also massage and touch the mother's abdominal area, although many only occasionally feel the baby while it is inside the womb. Frequent massage of the baby prior to birth helps the father to relate to the pregnancy experience and brings him closer to both the child and mother.

At the age of 5 or 6 a child usually begins to have the digital dexterity necessary to begin massaging their parents. Parents should encourage their child to do so. They should also be sure to respond with reassuring sighs and to offer the child compliments when a technique has been mastered. Too many children are brought up

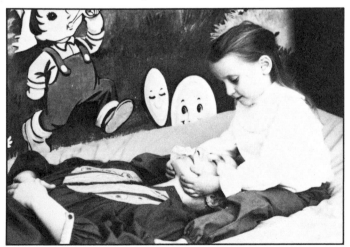

with little or no responsibility. As a result, they develop the attitude that whatever they need or desire will come to them with no effort on their part. Often they carry these unhealthy attitudes with them into adulthood. Massage is an excellent way to teach children that they can actively contribute to Mom and Dad's health and happiness.

Siblings, too, should be taught the techniques of massage. The more they exchange massages with each other, the better they will understand

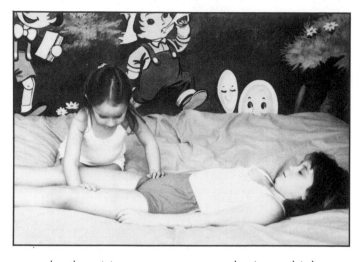

each other. Massage encourages sharing, which in turn promotes greater communication, builds trust and deepens the love between siblings, diminishing sibling rivalry.

Children, like adults, have physical and emotional complaints. When a child comes home after an upsetting day at school, what does a parent do instinctively to calm the child? Often a parent places the child's head in the hollow of the shoulder, then holds the back of the child's head or strokes the center of the child's back between the shoulder blades. The hollow of the adult's shoulder is touching the forehead frontal-eminence stress points of the child. The point on the back of the child's head corresponds to the adrenal glands, and contact there helps to relieve the tension produced by the upsetting events of the day. The neuro-lymphatic massage points for the emotional center of the brain are located in the center of the back. Intuitively the parent has touched all the correct points. The only problem is generally these points are not touched long enough or in a therapeutically effective way. Instead of giving a child an aspirin, parents should learn to stimulate the points that correspond to the child's complaints.

Minor illnesses respond quickly and easily to massage. With the knowledge gained from this book, a parent will be able to use massage and pressure points to bring about a speedy recovery in the child. Sore throats, colds, lung afflictions, earaches, toothaches, diarrhea and constipation are some of the common ailments that a parent can help a child overcome. Regular massage will also decrease a child's susceptibility to infections and improve the functioning of internal organs. It should also be remembered that children respond to massage much faster than most adults.

Equally important is the function of massage when a child is seriously ill and the parents, often totally frustrated, wish they could do something to help cure or improve the condition. This brings to mind the case of a newly married couple whose first baby was born with a hole in the heart. The doctors were uncertain as to whether the condition would improve. If it did, the doctors estimated it would take at least a year, and probably more. Frightened, helpless and miserable, the parents did not want simply to sit back and wait to see what would happen. Instead, they began using Touch for Health techniques to strengthen the baby's health. Within six months the hole had closed. The doctors were surprised, for they had never seen such a large hole close so quickly. The parents felt duly exultant, for they had helped to close the hole in their baby's heart. They had also turned agonizing months of helpless waiting into hopeful months of patient helping.

Massaging, holding or applying pressure to the points that correspond to a child's defective organ enables parents to feel helpful, and surely they are, for improved energy, blood and lymphatic circulation always helps an organ to function better and repair itself. It is understood, of course, that some illnesses are incurable; it is truly surprising to discover that most conditions can be improved through correct stimulation of the points associated with the organ involved.

Regular massage also helps a child to mature more readily and cope more effectively with social pressures and expectations. Children who grow up receiving massage tend not to experience major behavioral problems. And the severity of pre-existing behavioral problems for those children who did not receive massage throughout childhood may be lessened by beginning a regular massage program. Furthermore, massage can improve a child's perception of depth, thickness, texture and shape, in order to develop perceptive abilities at an age earlier than the childhood norm. Touch and massage can increase a child's I.Q., and what parent would not want a more intelligent daughter or son?

4) WHY SELF-MASSAGE?

Self-massage is infrequently utilized and greatly misunderstood. Most people have never heard of it, and those who have do not understand the extent of its benefits. Self-massage enhances an understanding of the body, and thus enables you to interpret your body signals with greater skill. The ability to translate your body signals into bodily needs can correct a disturbance long before it develops into a serious illness and can save you much pain and suffering.

Self-massage is a must for everyone. It is useful at any age, but self-help through massage is especially rewarding for older people who live alone. There will always be times when you need a massage and no one is available to administer it. Even if you live with someone, you will not always feel free to ask your partner for help. With the knowledge you obtain from this book, you can improve your physical health and psychological well-being.

Your health may benefit in many ways through self-massage. It can release blockages to improve the flow of your vital energies. It will develop your awareness of your skeletal and muscular systems enabling you to increase flexibility, and revitalize your constitution. The more you

learn about your body through self-massage, the greater your ability will be to improve its condition, and keep illness and pain out of your life.

Utilization of the proper points at the correct times can improve organic functions. To improve digestion, for example, you should do the stomach, pancreas, liver, gall bladder and small intestine points before and after meals. If you have just indulged in a greasy meal, by massaging the liver and gall bladder points you can help your body cope with the excess intake of fat. Don't fool yourself, however; fatty and fried foods are harmful. Do not assume that by assisting your liver and gall bladder each time you eat a fatty meal, you can undo all harm. This advice is meant to help you through only an occasional cheat. Self-massage can also be utilized to help organs that are not operating efficiently, as in cases of diabetes, heart problems or a weak bladder. By stimulating the correct points several times daily, you can vastly improve the function of the affected organ.

Take time to help your body. There are many ways you can help your vital organs. Let's say you're painting your house and the paint fumes become rather overpowering. It would make good sense, and provide relief, if you massaged your lung lymphatic points. Your liver, too, could use some assistance in coping with the extra load of toxins. You could also massage general circulation points.

Help is only as far away as your own hands in the event of household accidents. Should you hit your thumb with a hammer, you would instinctively hold it, squeeze it or suck on it. Such measures would make your thumb feel a little better, but an understanding of meridians, or energy pathways, would enable you to handle the accident more effectively. You would know that the lung meridian ends in your thumb, and that by pressing and massaging the origin of this meridian, which is located in the chest near the shoulder, you could relieve the pain and help your thumb to heal faster.

Self-massage also helps to firm or build up the muscles of your body. You can tone or develop major muscles of your body by using the corresponding points for the muscles you wish to

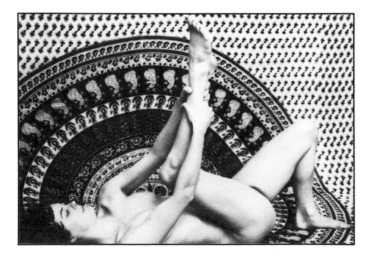

improve. By doing the points before and after you exercise, you can alert your body and brain to which muscles in particular you want to shape up.

If you often feel tired and lacking in energy, stimulation of your adrenal and brain points will provide a quick, safe pick-me-up. The energy boost you receive from massage, unlike caffeine and drugs, has no harmful side-effects. If, on the other hand, you are having trouble sleeping at night, sedation of your adrenal glands and holding your frontal eminence points will induce sleep in five minutes. Dangerous over-the-counter drugs are unnecessary.

Self-massage techniques will enable you to overcome tension instead of allowing it to overcome you. Traumatic events will no longer shatter you physically and emotionally. A telephone call bringing bad news, for instance, does not have to be debilitating. You probably have noticed many people place their hands on their foreheads in times of great stress. You have probably done it yourself. The neuro-vascular holding points that connect to the emotional center in the brain are located on the frontal eminence of the forehead. More by instinct than knowledge, you try to touch these correct holding points. With knowledge as well as instinct, however, you hold these points correctly and for the necessary length of time. The intensity of the traumatic experience would diminish, and you would become calmer, more rational and better able to cope. Some types of depression can also be controlled by utilizing the frontal eminence neuro-vascular holding points on a regular basis. Generally, self-massage can prevent accumulated daily psychological stresses from developing into a serious physical or emotional illness.

If you are extremely busy and don't have the time for self-massage, try incorporating some of the techniques into each day's shower or bath. By the end of one week you will have stimulated all your major organs. Your body will be grateful for the extra help. It has a big job coping with all the tension and toxins in the world today.

Many people tell me that self-massage is not as satisfying as being massaged by someone else, and so why bother? Well, I can't deny it. Lying down for one hour and receiving a massage is far more pleasant than having to do it yourself. Nevertheless, some physical manipulation is preferable to none, as is feeling healthy and fit to being sickly and tired. No one knows your body as well as you. With some knowledge of massage and your instincts as your guide, you will know better than anyone else where and how you need to be touched. You will also know how much pressure to apply without causing pain. Much of the feeling of pain is really fear of pain. When you are in control of the pressure, you eliminate the fear and can therefore press harder than a massage therapist might. In some instances, increased pressure brings faster and greater relief. Remember, too, that once the mechanical process of learning the techniques is accomplished, you are free to focus on the sensations emanating from the point of contact and to increase the pleasures of self-massage.

Massaging yourself is a very positive statement. You love yourself. You think you deserve the time and attention, and you give it to yourself. While it seems natural and right to help others, caring for oneself seems somehow indulgent. We have been conditioned from childhood to believe that being good to ourselves is wrong. Loving ourselves is considered a worse offense. It's time to stop perpetuating this fallacy. If you can't be good to yourself, how can someone else be good to you! If you don't love yourself, who will love you? Finding and keeping love or friendship begins with you and your ability to love yourself, and then with your capacity to love someone else.

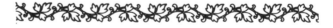

CHAPTER III

What You Need To Know For Best Results

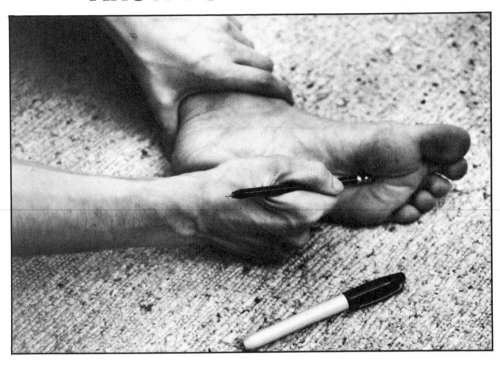

1) PREPARATIONS & ACCESSORIES

a) GENERAL PREPARATIONS & ACCESSORIES

Silence your telephone. If the telephone rings while you are receiving a massage, it will jangle your nervous system. It will wake you if you are sleeping and interrupt your flow of communication if you are not. Take your phone off the hook, or else turn down the ring and either cover the phone with a pillow or put it into a dresser drawer or closet. If you have an answering machine, switch it on and turn down all volume settings. If you have a jack, unplug it. Do as you please, but be sure to take care of this important matter. During massage, the telephone is an unwelcome intrusion.

Do not disturb. Place a "do not disturb" sign on your door to discourage unexpected visits from friends or neighbors. On it state the time you will be available, and if you have a doorman, tell him during which hours you will *not* be receiving. The time you set aside for massage is special. Do not allow interruptions.

Turn off glaring lights. Subtle lighting is a must. Bright lights strain the eyes and make it difficult to relax. When you become experienced at massage, try doing it in the dark. Without your eyesight your sense of touch becomes much more acute.

Control temperature. Air-conditioning is fine for the doer during the summer months. The receiver, however, will probably feel cold, as body temperature drops during a massage. A fan directed at the doer is ideal, for its breeze will only indirectly reach the receiver and will be deflected enough not to cause a chill. In the winter, when additional heat is required, do not use a space heater. Its intense heat can make the doer faint. Also, one part of the receiver's body is likely to be burning hot and the rest uncomfortably chilled.

An electric heater is dangerous because sheets, carpets and even flesh can easily be burned. Use an electric blanket whenever the receiver is likely to be cold. A receiver who feels chilled or cold will become tense and find the massage most unpleasant. Neither receiver nor doer benefits from a discomforting massage. If the doer exposes only the part of the body being massaged, the receiver will remain warm, relaxed and secure under the electric blanket.

Control drafts. A slight draft is harmless to the doer, but it can be quite chilling to the receiver. Drafts decrease the pleasure of the massage, diminish its benefits and can cause stiff or cramped muscles.

Incense creates a relaxing atmosphere . If you enjoy the fragrance of burning incense, use it. If, however, you start to sneeze, you may be allergic to it.Teary eyes and difficulty breathing are also allergic reactions.Incense is not essential,but the fragrance is conducive to relaxation and enjoyment.

Massage on a mat on the floor. A 1¹/₂-inch foam mat covered with a sheet is ideal, but if you do not want to invest in a mat, the blanket method is adequate. If one of your floors is padded and carpeted, all you need is two blankets. Fold each blanket into thirds. Stack one on top of the other. Spread a sheet over the blankets, and you've got it. Two blankets, stacked on a carpeted and padded floor, usually provide enough padding for the receiver's back and enough cushioning for the doer's knees. Remember, if the doer is not comfortable, that discomfort is transmitted to the receiver, and the pleasure and benefits are diminished for both. Do not give a massage on a mattress or futon. Instead of penetrating the receiver, most of the force of your pressure will be absorbed by the mattress. Furthermore, the receiver will become increasingly more conscious of the doer's every move, and the massage itself will become rocky and distracting. It is also quite easy for the doer to fall onto the receiver, as it is difficult to keep your balance on a mattress.

Prepare an extra blanket. If you do not own an electric blanket, keep a soft blanket handy in the event that the receiver gets cold. For some people a sheet is sufficient, but most require a blanket for warmth part way through the massage. If the room can't be adequately heated, you may need two blankets for the receiver. Fold each blanket in four. Cover the receiver's torso with one blanket, and use the other for the legs and feet. Expose only that part of the body you are massaging in order to guarantee the receiver's comfort.

For the sake of clarity all photographs depict the receiver under ideal temperature conditions, thereby rendering a sheet or cover unnecessary.

Music soothes and relaxes. Music played softly in the background encourages relaxation. Loud music, however, distracts rather than soothes. Excellent selections of music, recorded for the express purpose of relaxing overly stimulated nervous systems, are available on tape. Some people find recordings of sea sounds particularly effective. Others prefer tapes of bird calls, which can lull the receiver's mind with the tranquil sounds of the country on a bright sunny day. I don't advise listening to music that is accompanied by lyrics, because lyrics tend to keep the mind focused rather than allowing it to free-associate. Select the music of your choice, and have the tapes or records ready to be played prior to beginning the massage. See page 184 for suggestions on the purchase of appropriate music.

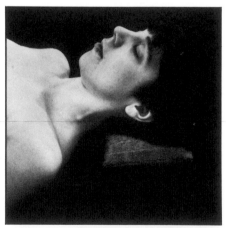

Raise the head with a pillow.

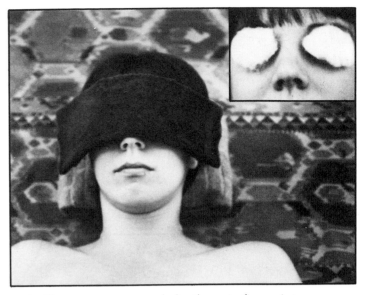

Raise the head with a pillow. Place a thin 1 to 2 inch pillow under the receiver's head. When the receiver is lying in the supine position, the head tilts back slightly and pinches the first few cervical vertebrae. Elevation of the head releases this pressure from the affected vertebrae. It thereby encourages the body to relax more readily and to be more receptive to the benefits of massage. If you don't have a thin pillow, use a towel folded several times. Prepare the pillow or towel prior to beginning the massage, and keep it within easy reach so that you can insert it without any distraction under the receiver's head.

Raise the receiver's legs while lying supine and prone. Place one folded bed pillow under each

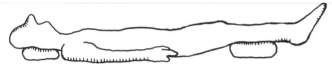

of the receiver's legs. Lying flat on the back puts a strain on the lower back. Since the receiver is supine during more than half the massage, low back strain or pain can easily result. People who suffer from back pain will almost always develop some discomfort during the massage if their legs are not raised. Even those who don't will find that their lower back begins to ache from lying supine too long. Raising the legs reduces the arch of the lower back and thus removes the strain on the muscles of the lower back. Use the same pillows

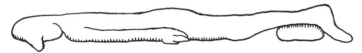

under the ankles while the receiver is lying prone. Not only will back tension be lessened, but also the feet will rest more comfortably on the mat.

Relieve eye-strain. Place cotton balls soaked in witch hazel, or in a cold solution of the herb eyebright, over the closed eyes. Drape a folded towel over the eyes and forehead. The folded towel serves both to cover the frontal eminence tension points and to keep the cotton balls in place. If you prefer to use eyebright, which can be purchased in most health food stores, prepare the solution by steeping one teaspoon of the herb in one cup of

boiling water, covered, for three to five mintues. Use only a fresh solution of eyebright. Refrigeration keeps a solution of eyebright fresh for two to three days. Chill the eyebright or witch hazel prior to application. Be sure to state that you are placing cold cotton balls over the eyes in order to prepare the receiver for the cold sensation.

Oil the back. You may use a small amount of oil on the back prior to beginning Back Technique #4, which is described in Chapter IV. It is not necessary, although some people feel a massage is incomplete unless they are oiled. In any case, use the oil sparingly. Work it well into the skin with upward or downward long, stroking motions. The back must not be oily or slippery when you begin Technique #4. Do not use oil on any other part of the body, as oiling interferes with pressure techniques. Massaging oil into the back does help to release some of the superficial tension stored in the muscles. This stroking motion, known as effleurage, also significantly improves venous and lymph circulation. The following oils are excellent: coconut, safflower, sesame, olive and almond, or any combination of these.

Remove jewelry. Jewelry can interfere with massaging techniques by scratching the receiver's skin. As this would be an unexpected, unpleasant and unwelcome experience for the receiver, play it safe by removing bracelets, watches and rings.

Short finger nails are important. Nails that extend beyond the tips of the fingers are too long for comfortable massage.

Clean hands are a must. As you will be touching the receiver's eyes and your fingers will be in the receiver's ears, clean hands are an absolute MUST. Many unpleasant conditions can be communicated via the hands. To avoid the possibility of any embarrassing situations, begin every massage with freshly washed hands and well-scrubbed nails. Clean hands also allow for greater sensitivity.

To be or not to be nude? If you are massaging your lover, it is sometimes very nice to be nude along with your partner. The reason is not at all sexual. Removing the clothing barrier allows both of you to relax more readily. Equally exposed and vulnerable, you can more easily share the inti - macy of massage and achieve a feeling of oneness.

Wear loose clothing. Tight pants or shirts will make your experience as the doer most unpleasant. Avoid cutting off the circulation to any part of the body by wearing loose, comfortable clothing.

Don't forget the cold water wash. After completing a massage, it is an excellent idea to rub your hands together vigorously under *cold* water and allow the water to run from above your elbows down your forearm. Any negative energy that may have seeped from the receiver's body into your hands can be released in this manner. You will feel the difference, and you will also prevent unwanted energy from entering your body.

b) SPECIAL CONSIDERATIONS FOR MASSAGING CHILDREN

Draft & temperature control are especially important for young infants and children. If the possiblity exists for the child to experience a chill, massage the child in soft, loose, comfortable clothing.

Children new to massage are sometimes fidgety. Until the child adjusts to being handled in this manner, a teddy bear or soft cuddly friend will help. Initially, the child will fondle the toy, but will soon ignore it and enjoy the massage.

c) SPECIAL CONSIDERATIONS FOR SELF-MASSAGE

Tools can help. A ball point pen with an eraser or a thick marker pen with a rounded end can be useful when massaging the bottom of the foot. Unless your thumbs are exceptionally strong, they may tire or ache. These tools will enable you to apply firm pressure and experience maximum

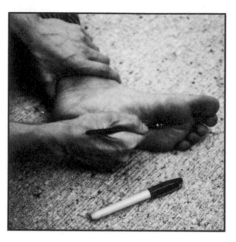

penetration with the least effort. Keep your tools clean. Your natural oils, as they accumulate on the tools, can make it dangerous, because your grip may slip while you are applying pressure. The result could be a painful experience. If you don't like the idea of using a foreign object, alternately use your thumbs and knuckles to apply pressure.

Loofa sponge. If you massage yourself in the tub or like to take a bath immediately after a massage, a loofa sponge rub is a great way both to end your massage and to improve circulation.

Pillows. Keep several pillows handy. You may need one or more of the pillows to help you assume a position comfortably.

d) SPECIAL CONSIDERATIONS FOR A QUICKIE MASSAGE

Spread a sheet on a carpeted and padded floor, turn down the telephone, dim the lights, and begin. Perhaps you have switched on some soothing music to help release tension, and the receiver may have undressed. Neither music nor nudity, however, is essential for a quickie massage. Time is. In Japan many people enjoy the refreshment of a Shiatsu massage during a lunch break, when time is obviously limited. A quickie massage can change the mind of any partner or friend who says, "I just can't go out tonight, I'm too tired." It will take you 15-25 minutes to convince your partner otherwise, for that is how quickly the Magic of Massage works.

2) PROPER FRAME OF MIND FACILITATES MOVEMENT OF BODY ENERGIES

Set all worries and thoughts aside. Remember that a worried or preoccupied mind cannot give the all that is necessary for a magical and therapeutically effective massage. The receiver will undoubtedly benefit to some degree from an absent-mindedly administered massage, but why settle for less? If you're going to give a massage, give it. Be there.

If you are one of those people who doesn't feel quite right unless your mind is active with worry or thought, try thinking about helping the receiver to relax and enjoy the massage. You can worry in double time, once the massage is over. Chances are greater, however, that after a few weeks of giving and receiving massage, you won't feel quite so compelled to worry. Massage on a regular basis does wonders for compulsive worriers, because the magic of massage calms not only the body but also the mind.

Keep your mind free and clear from mundane thoughts. While some people are given to excessive worry and gnawing anxiety, others are plagued by the trivial and mundane. Free your mind of lists and chores, of shopping or laundry that must be done, of floors that need washing, of lawns that should have been cut last week. Be there, with the receiver and the massage. An uncluttered mind effects a better massage.

Fill your mind and body with caring and compassion. At least fifty percent of the success of massage is determined by how much you, as the doer, want to help. Your only concern should be the well-being of the receiver. Your compassion will encourage the receiver to release tension and to enjoy a far more effective massage. What you give is reflected in what you receive. If your mind is focused exclusively on the receiver, you will drop your defenses and magically share in the benefits of the massage along with the receiver.

Breathing is important. When massaging yourself or someone else, allow yourself at least one minute before beginning the massage to regulate your breathing. Slower and slightly deeper than normal breaths will put you in touch with the "now" of the experience and will enable you to give a more effective massage. Do not inhale or exhale so deeply that breathing becomes an effort. Deep, but relaxed breathing is the secret. Don't force huge quantities of air into or out of your lungs. Simply inhale completely, then exhale completely. Little by little you will begin to relax. The depth of your inhalations and exhalations will automatically increase, because your diaphragm will have become more and more relaxed. Focus on your breathing. Focused breathing quiets the body and mind at the same time that it increases awareness of physical sensations. Deep breathing also oxygenates the blood. A body that is deprived of its fair share of oxygen experiences fatigue more rapidly than one accustomed to the rewards of deep breathing. Unfortunately, most of us are shallow breathers, as foul-smelling air, coupled with tension, discourages full breathing. Over a period of years, however, shallow breathing only intensifies that tension and increases the chances of illness. So, remain subliminally focused on your breathing pattern. Keep it slow and a little deeper than usual.

Keep your body relaxed. If your body is not relaxed while you massage, you will become tired and tense. You won't enjoy the experience, nor will the receiver. Consequently, both of you may shy away from the routine of massage. Hang loose! Giving a massage should be a pleasant experience. Allow your head to float freely on your neck, and keep your shoulders relaxed, not tense and raised up to your ears. Keep your back as straight as possible and free from abnormal concave or convex curves. Make frequent mental checks to maintain your relaxed posture.

Know what you are massaging. Do not think of massage as an application of pressure only to the skin. You want to reach the core of the receiver. Think penetration—penetration to the bones' very marrow, to the vital centers of the organs and to the core of the nervous system. Be aware that to penetrate does not mean to cause pain. Focus your attention on the point of contact. What does it feel like? Is the point soft, hard, hot, cold, raised, hollow, active or dead? Do you feel energy radiating from the pressure point? Allow your instincts to dictate how much pressure to apply.

What is the receiver's frame of mind? The receiver should also focus attention on the pressure applied to each point. Focusing on the contact points helps to keep the receiver's mind free of extraneous worries and thoughts. This kind of concentration will often induce the receiver to fall asleep very soon after the beginning of the massage. The receiver must be submissive, must allow the doer to penetrate to the very core of her/his being. Above all, the receiver must be willing to receive the magic of massage.

Focus your attention. If the pressure point or massage technique corresponds to a particular organ, focus your attention on that organ. Try to imagine the organ's location in the body, and try to visualize its shape and size. With a little practice, thorough concentration and a lot of desire, both the receiver and the doer will be able to feel the energy moving into and through the organ being dealt with. Furthermore, the energy, blood and nutrients will reach their destination with greater ease when you focus your attention.

Execute Penetration with slow, sure strokes. Once you have made contact with a pressure point, penetration must be slow and easy. Never poke or dig unexpectedly into the receiver. When applying pressure, begin very gently and gradually increase your pressure to approximately half the receiver's capacity. When you are certain the receiver is comfortable, slowly proceed to apply the remainder of the pressure. Massage and pressure techniques must be executed with patience and without haste. Fast or energetic movements will jar the receiver out of the placid state you have worked so hard to achieve. Remember, your aim is to relax and soothe. As your confidence, or lack of it, will be picked up intuitively by the receiver, work slowly, easily and surely.

Establish a regular rhythm. A predictable rhythm calms the mind and relaxes the body. The application of pressure or massage in a hypnotically repetitive rhythm disposes the mind to ignore all but what is being done to the body. Keep your rhythms slow, as fast rhythms fail to relax effectively. A slow, predictable rhythm will also facilitate the movement of body energies.

Close your eyes. By closing your eyes, you eliminate your sense of sight and heighten your sense of touch. The more intense your touch, the more compassionate and magical will be your massage. Until recently, all practitioners of massage in Japan were blind. Not only did this marvelous custom create work and a meaningful existence for blind individuals, but also the receivers experienced an extraordinarily sensitive and compassionate massage.

Music calms the mind. If it is difficult for you to achieve the proper frame of mind for massage, music can be a useful tool to calm and soothe the mind. Choose music that both you and the receiver enjoy, though classical, jazz or cosmic sounds are most conducive to massage. Tapes are better than records. Tapes can easily be reversed with one hand, while the other remains in constant contact with the receiver. Keep the tape recorder close at hand, so that you don't have to break this contact. If possible, record some of your favorite music on a 45-minute tape. Tapes offering forty-five mintues of cosmic sounds are available especially for massage. Music without lyrics is preferable, and keep the volume low. Music should enhance and complement the massage, not dominate it.

Chanting clears your mind and relaxes your body. If you don't have tapes or records suitable for massage, chanting can effectively clear your mind and relax your body. If you don't know how to chant, hum random notes. Do not feel inhibited. Let your instincts dictate whether you should hum a low or high note. Begin humming the note immediately after you have inhaled deeply, and continue it as long as you can exhale comfortably. The sound and vibration of the hum should come from the abdomen or lower chest, not from the throat, mouth or nose. If the sounds and vibrations emanate from these upper regions of your body, you are tense and need to make a conscious effort to relax and lower the hum to the abdominal area. Don't hum a familiar tune, as it will bring intrusive associations to mind. The notes you hum should be random and inspirational. Let them reflect your feelings and needs. Vary the pitch and duration of each sound. Chanting can create a strong feeling of oneness between you and the receiver that will encourage the release of energy and increase the benefits of massage.

Prepare for unexpected disturbances.
If you have attended to all the preparations and accessories listed in this section of the book, you will begin the massage calm, relaxed and confident. Sensing your readiness, the receiver will more easily submit to your touch and the magic of massage.

Proper frame of mind for self-massage. In self-massage you are both the doer and the receiver. As the doer, you must learn to function without much thought or effort. Several practice massages should enable you to master the techniques sufficiently, and the actual doing of the massage will cease to command your attention. As the receiver, you are primarily the experiencer. Focus your attention more on the physical sensations of your self-massage than on its technical execution. The more conscious you are of sensual responses, the greater will be your pleasure and the more fully realized your benefits. Practice makes perfect. Self-massage can be almost as rewarding and fulfilling as being massaged by someone else, if you maintain the proper frame of mind and allow the magic of massage to flow through your hands.

Learn to develop X-ray vision. Study the anatomical diagrams. (Terminology is irrelevant.)Then close your eyes and try to visualize them in detail. Practice this frequently, five minutes at a time. Soon you will be able to see into the body you are massaging. (If possible, study a skeleton to improve the three dimensionality of your vision.)

3)HOW TO GIVE A MASSAGE WITHOUT FEELING FATIGUED

It's easy to give a massage without feeling fatigued by the process. You simply have to know the tricks of the trade. These tricks or rules can be applied to all massage, be it massage for children, the family pet, someone else or yourself. It will require some discipline, at first, to learn the tricks, but if you practice them assiduously and keep regular check on yourself, you will soon be subconsciously assuming the correct posture, positioning and angle of penetration. Without effort you will be allowing the magic of massage to flow without interruption.

Assume the correct posture for the technique you are using. Be sure to study the photographs and text accompanying each technique. Try to assume exactly the posture shown in the photographs or described in the text. These postures are time-tested and offer maximum comfort for most people. If for some reason you are unable to assume the recommended posture, work out one that is comfortable and practical for you. Keep in mind, however, that you must not be hunched while you work. Try also to position yourself so that you are perpendicular to the surface to which you are applying pressure.

Comfort is of utmost importance. If at any time your position ceases to be comfortable, you must alter your posture. Otherwise, your discomfort will be transmitted to the receiver, and the massage will be a less pleasurable experience for both of you. The trick is to change positions without disturbing the receiver. NEVER move suddenly or jump up quickly. And do not take your hands off the receiver's body while trying to assume a different, more comfortable position. Abrupt and disruptive movements break down the bond between the doer and receiver, and five or six such disturbances could defeat the purpose of the massage. Your aim is to create an atmosphere of serenity, confidence and mutual trust. To maintain it requires that changes in position be gradual and

subtle. For example, if you are applying pressure and suddenly find that you are intolerably uncomfortable, begin to shift your position inch by inch to one more comfortable. You must know in advance which position you wish to assume and *gradually* move into it. Do not move while you are applying pressure. Instead, alternate movement with application of pressure. Press, then move a little; press, then move a little. Follow this procedure until the desired change of position is achieved. All movement and any alteration of position throughout the process of massage should combine grace with ease and subtlety in order not to disturb the receiver. For massage to work its magic, your every move must be magically imperceptible.

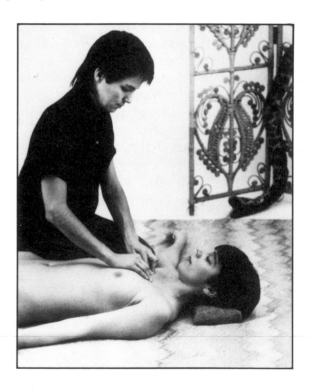

Keep your spine erect. Do not allow your back to sag. The upper back must be straight and relaxed, not hunched forward. The lower back must be as close to flat as possible. Avoid a concave depression in the small of the back, which results from the protrusion of the buttocks. As you massage, periodically check the orientation of your spine. If you are slouching or arched, straighten your spine slowly, but do not disturb the receiver.

Keep your shoulders loose and relaxed. Massaging with tense shoulders will cause much discomfort in a matter of minutes. To keep shoulders loose and relaxed is a little tricky at first, but practice will soon enable you to master that technique. Begin by letting your shoulders hang

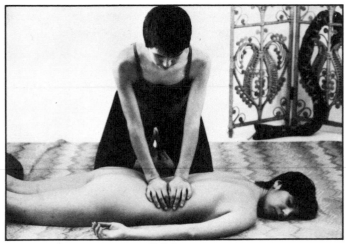

CORRECT

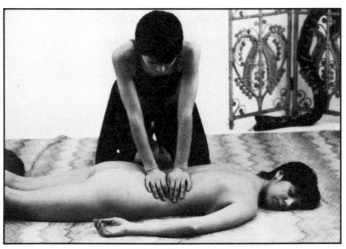

INCORRECT

loose. Concentrate, while you massage, on keeping your shoulders in this loose position. I don't mean by this that you should tense them in order to maintain their lowered position, but rather that you should concentrate on allowing them to hang low and loose. Focus on keeping your shoulders in this relaxed position as you work.

Do not use muscle power to apply pressure. When applying thumb pressure, use your body weight and your hara, not your shoulder muscle

power. Imagine a magical force surging up from your torso, then streaming down your arms and into the receiver. Feel your strength rising up from within you. Do not rely on muscle power. Unless you are muscularly an extremely powerful person, you will soon exhaust your strength and tire. Try to develop your ability to massage from your hara. Hara is the Japanese word for the center of the energy of your body. The Japanese believe that when you function from your hara, all things are more easily accomplished, and I have certainly found this true in my own experience. Your hara is located one and a half inches below your navel.

Do not abuse your thumbs. Many of the pressure techniques require the use of your thumbs.

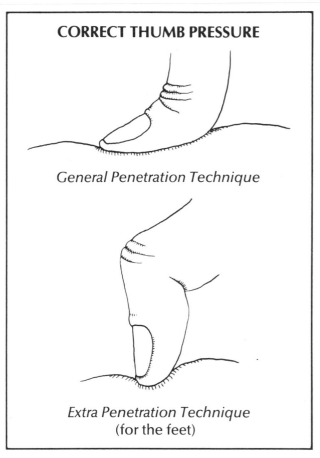

CORRECT THUMB PRESSURE

General Penetration Technique

Extra Penetration Technique
(for the feet)

If at any time you experience a shooting pain or a very tired sensation in your thumbs, switch to the use of your fingers, knuckles, elbows or knees. The heel of your foot and the heel of your hand are also useful tools.

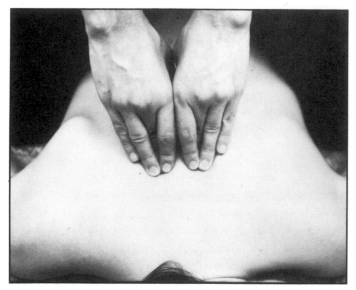

Your fingers can be used in much the same manner as your thumbs, because they, too, are soft and padded. Use your middle finger braced by the two fingers on either side of it. Remember to keep your shoulders loose and your spine erect as you work. There is a tendency to lose the correct posture when using a different technique.

When employing the knuckles, it is important to remember that much less pressure is required, because the knuckles, unlike the thumbs, are not well padded. Practice knuckle pressure on the re-

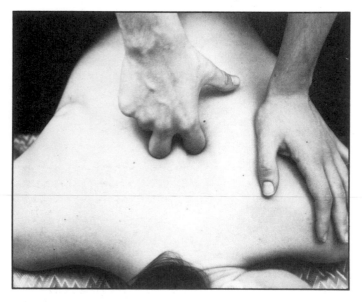

ceiver prior to beginning your first massage, so that you are aware of the extent of the receiver's tolerance for this technique. Knuckle pressure, like any other, is to be enjoyed and should not hurt. Keep a close watch on the receiver's face. The facial expressions will let you know whether the pressure you are applying is appropriate or not. If at any time you are uncertain about the amount of pressure, quietly ask your partner if it feels all right.

Elbows can be used with as much compassion and can be equally as effective as thumbs. Elbows are, however, very bony, so great care must be taken when you are using them in massage. If your frame is small and you are working on a

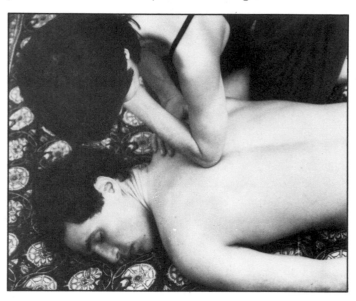

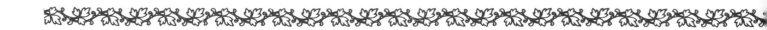

large person, your elbows can be especially useful along the spine. You will achieve excellent results with a minimal expenditure of effort and energy, and thereby conserve your strength for the rest of the massage. Apply pressure with your elbow to the tsubos, or pressure points, along one side of the spine, while resting the hand of your other arm on the receiver's back to provide a comforting touch. Repeat the same procedure for the other side.

Knees, too, can be useful tools. The knee can be applied to a specific pressure point and at the same time cover a general area. The most important thing to remember about this very sensitive addition to your repertoire of massage techniques is that the most prominent bony protrusion is the

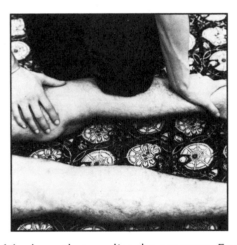

part of the knee that applies the pressure. Focus your attention on this protrusion as you work, so that you will know when you have applied enough pressure. Feel how deep it is penetrating. Only the bony protrusion is the tool. The rest of the knee is along for the ride.

The heels of your feet are useful in several instances. For example, if you're feeling a strain in your thumbs and the receiver's feet have yet to be massaged, use your feet. Walk on the bottom of your partner's feet. Apply pressure to the same areas as you would with your thumbs. Rest most of your body weight on each of the reflex points for three to five seconds. Some people can enjoy more pressure than others, so be sure to ask the receiver if the pressure is comfortable. You will

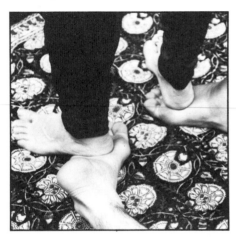

not be able to be quite as thorough working with your feet as with your thumbs, but you will be able to stimulate most of the reflex points. What you cannot reach with your feet can be completed afterwards with your thumbs or fingers. Maintain your balance with a chair if you feel you might fall. The heels can also be useful on the shoulders, the back of the legs and the buttocks. Always observe the receiver for reactions of pain.

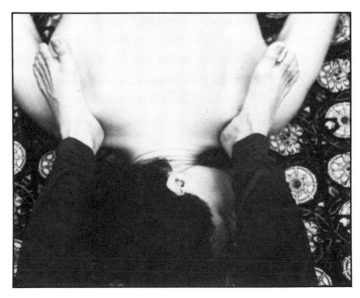

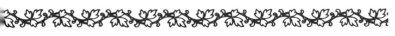

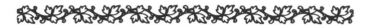

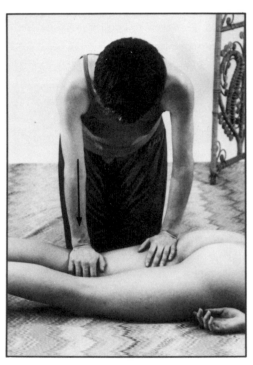

Positioning is important. Try to duplicate the positions illustrated in the text. These positions have been tested and proven to be comfortable and practical. Do not stretch to implement a technique. Do not work off balance.

The correct angle of penetration is important. Try as much as possible to apply pressure from directly above the area you are addressing. The angle of penetration should be perpendicular to the surface receiving the pressure. Your body weight will fall naturally onto the tsubo, and no muscle power will be needed.

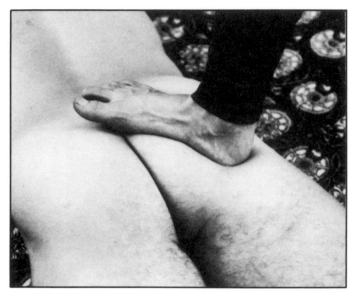

The heel of your hand can be used for meridian tracing and specific point pressure. The entire surface of the heel of your hand is perfect for Technique #63, Upper Arm Lung Meridian Tracing. The bony protrusion at the wrist provides an

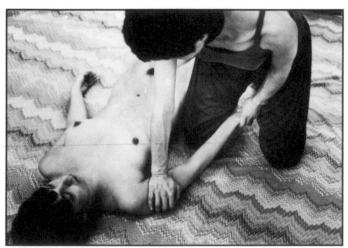

excellent tool for applying pressure to specific tsubos. Simply direct the force of the pressure down your arm, into this bony protrusion and into the receiver's body. Keep your hand relaxed as you work.

4)WHAT IS AN ECLECTIC MASSAGE?

A well known dictionary definition of eclectic is: "*Adj.* 1. selecting; choosing from various sources. 2. made up of what is selected from different sources. 3. not following any one system, as of philosophy, medicine, etc., but selecting and using what are considered the best elements of all systems . . ."

Acupuncture Meridian Therapy without the use of a needle, which is also known as Acupressure, Acupuncture Holding/Pressure Point Therapy, Acu-therapy or Shiatsu, has been combined with Foot Reflexology, Touch for Health's Neurovascular Holding Points and Neuro-lymphatic Massage, Swedish Massage and some original material to produce an unusual system that integrates Eastern and Western approaches to body therapy. This book offers a new system of body maintenance and improvement, combining benefits from the most respected and effective disciplines in the field of physical health care. This system stimulates the body's own natural healing mechanism. Rather than directly effecting a cure, it encourages the body to do what it can to right a condition of ill health.

5)DISCIPLINES RELEVANT TO THIS SYSTEM OF ECLECTIC MASSAGE

The following pages highlight those aspects of the disciplines relevant to this system of eclectic massage that the author feels are most important for the reader's general knowledge. The information is by no means complete. For further information on any of the following disciplines, please refer to the Bibliography.

a) ACUPUNCTURE = acu(s)/needle + punctura/puncture

- A very thin needle penetrates the acupuncture points (tsubos), which are located along the meridians or energy pathway

- Penetration is shallow, no more than a few millimeters, and can be held for up to 30 minutes or longer

- Penetration executed efficiently results in little or no pain

- Meridians or energy pathways have been charted by modern electronic instruments

- Meridians are not only located on the surface of the body, as depicted in most drawings, but are also located deep within the body

- The meridian energy does not flow in a vessel, as does blood or lymph; therefore, the Western medical mind has had trouble accepting the ancient Eastern meridian theory, despite the fact that modern instruments have proven meridians do exist

- Many different theories attempt to explain how acupuncture works, but no one theory has found total acceptance

- It is important to remember that although Western medicine refuses to accept acupuncture into its mainstream, Eastern medicine continues to utilize acupuncture as a safe and effective method of anesthetizing patients during surgery. It also successfully treats many diseases and conditions with acupuncture

- Acupuncture relies on two basic methods for treating a health problem, the acupuncture of points close to the problem and the acupuncture of points distant from the problem

- The Western medical mind can more easily accept acupuncture of the *locus dolenti*, or points close to the problem, as a means of treatment, although acupuncture of distant points often proves more effective

- Acupuncture encourages the body's natural healing mechanism

- A total of fifty-nine meridians is commonly used in traditional Chinese acupuncture

- The twelve basic meridians and two other extra meridians, known as the governing and conception vessels, are the meridians of primary concern in this book

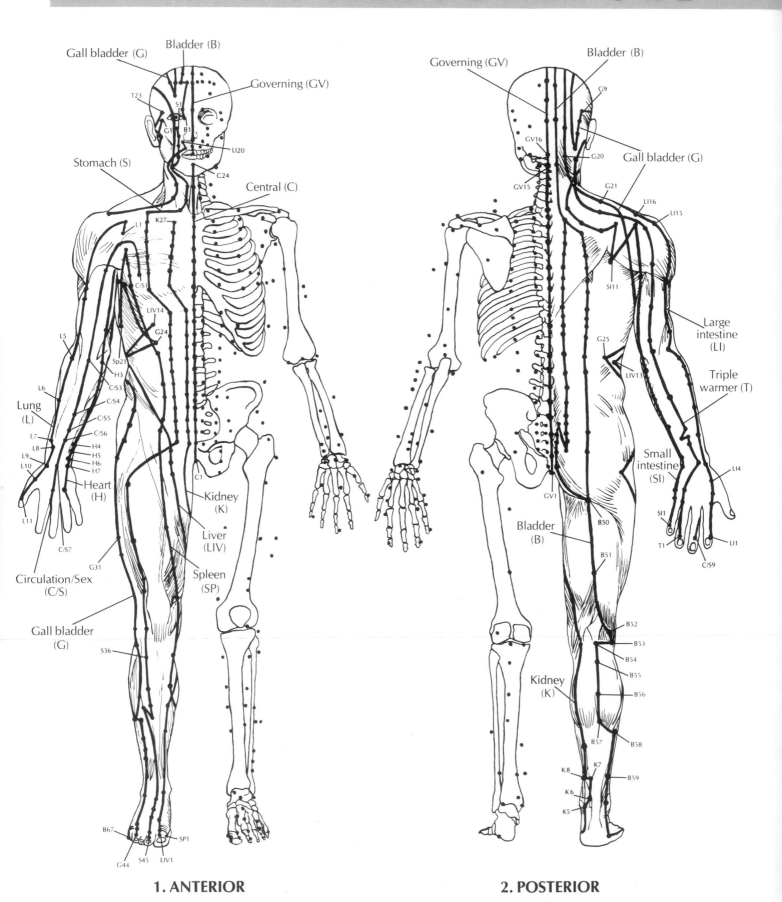

1. ANTERIOR

2. POSTERIOR

REFERENCE CHART

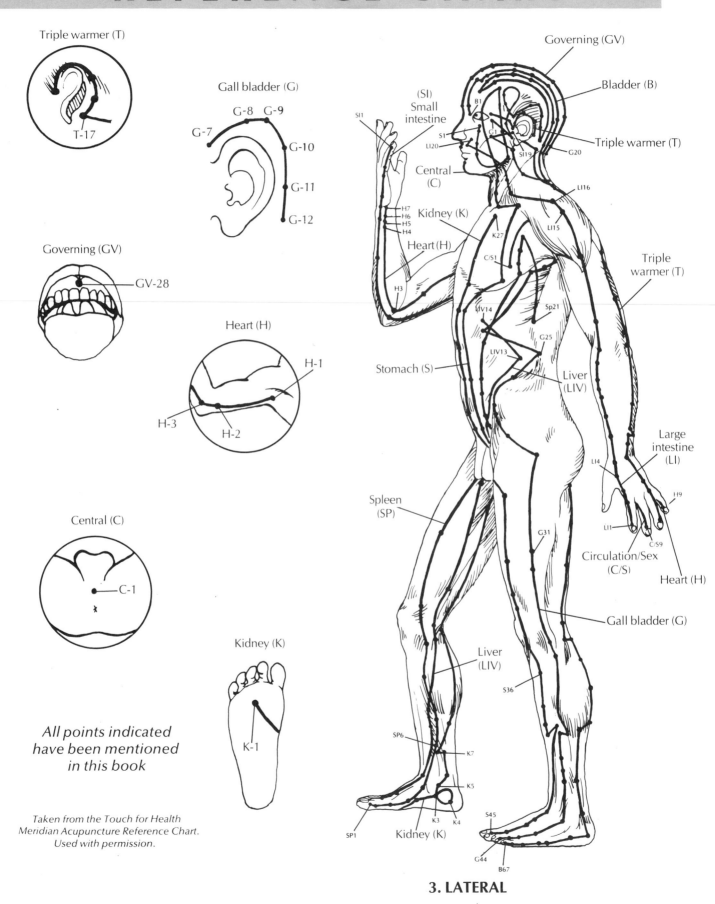

Triple warmer (T)

T-17

Gall bladder (G)

G-8 G-9
G-7
G-10
G-11
G-12

Governing (GV)

GV-28

Heart (H)

H-1
H-3
H-2

Central (C)

C-1

All points indicated
have been mentioned
in this book

Kidney (K)

K-1

Taken from the Touch for Health
Meridian Acupuncture Reference Chart.
Used with permission.

Governing (GV)
Bladder (B)
(SI)
Small intestine
Triple warmer (T)
SI1
B1
S1
LI20
G1
SI19
G20
Central (C)
LI16
Kidney (K)
H7
H6
H5
H4
K27
LI15
Heart (H)
C/S1
H3
Triple warmer (T)
LIV14
Sp21
G25
LIV13
Stomach (S)
Liver (LIV)
Large intestine (LI)
LI4
Spleen (SP)
LI1
H9
C/S9
Circulation/Sex (C/S)
Heart (H)
G31
Liver (LIV)
Gall bladder (G)
S36
SP6
K7
K5
SP1
K3 K4
Kidney (K)
S45
G44
B67

3. LATERAL

MERIDIAN	**ASSOCIATED ORGAN OR AILMENT	ASSOCIATED MUSCLES
Conception/ Central	Brain	Supraspinatus
Governing	Spine & Nervous System	Teres Major
Stomach	Stomach tension & insomnia sinus & allergies headaches	Pectoralis Major Clavicular Levator Scapula Neck Muscles Brachioradialis
Spleen	Spleen Pancreas infections & fevers anemia	Latissimus Dorsi Trapezius Opponens Pollicis Triceps
Heart	Heart	Subscapularis
Small Intestine	Small Intestine digestive disturbances low back pain knee problems	Quadriceps Abdominals
Bladder	Bladder ankle problems & flat feet bunions emotional strain arthritis	Peroneus Sacrospinalis Tibialis
Kidney	Kidney skin problems dark marks under the eyes great thirst low back pain heart conditions eye & ear problems	Psoas Upper Trapezius Iliacus
Heart Constrictor/ Circulation-Sex	general circulation sex organs menstrual problems, breast pain, menopause prostate problems impotency sciatic pain bladder conditions	Gluteus Medius & Maximus Adductors Piriformis
Triple Heater/ Triple Warmer	Thyroid Adrenals Pancreas sugar problems infections	Teres Minor Sartorius Gracilis Soleus Gastrocnemius

MERIDIAN	**ASSOCIATED ORGAN OR AILMENT	ASSOCIATED MUSCLES
Gall Bladder	digestion & Gall Bladder conditions	Anterior Deltoid Popliteus
Liver	Liver grey spots interfering with vision glaucoma lengthy headaches	Pectoralis Major Sternal Rhomboids
Lungs	Lungs all lung conditions	Anterior Serratus Coracobrachialis Deltoids Diaphragm
Large Intestine	Large Intestine all conditions pertaining to the large intestines painful breasts and chest during menstruation restlessness & exhaustion headaches	Fascia Lata Hamstrings Quadratus Lumborum

**Associated Organ or Ailment. These ailments related to the associated organ, as well as many others not listed above, can be improved or cured by acupuncture meridian therapy.

b) ACUPUNCTURE HOLDING/ PRESSURE POINTS

(Acupressure or Acu-therapy: Misnomers, because *acu-* means needle and no needles are used.)

- No needles are used in acupuncture holding/ pressure points

- Light finger contact is applied to the skin at the acupuncture points or tsubos for holding points and heavy pressure for pressure points

- As with acupuncture, repeated applications of the light or heavy finger contact are usually necessary to effect a cure or lessen symptoms

- The great advantage of acupuncture holding/ pressure points is that you can help yourself

- Some doctors and chiropractors are now teaching their patients the acupuncture holding/pressure points relevant to the patient's particular condition

- Holding points must be held for 20-30 seconds in order to elicit a reaction

- Touch for Health utilizes acupuncture holding points

- Shiatsu utilizes acupuncture pressure points

- Pressure points must be held for 3-10 seconds or up to one minute depending upon the severity of the condition

c) SHIATSU=
shi/fingers + atsu/pressure

- This discipline primarily utilizes thumb pressure which is applied to the tsubos

- Most shiatsu is based on the twelve basic and two extra ancient Chinese acupuncture meridians discussed above under ACUPUNCTURE, although some practitioners use other meridian systems as well

- The Japanese Ministry of Health and Welfare states that Shiatsu therapy can "correct internal malfunctioning, promote health, and treat specific diseases"

- Shiatsu pressure is firmer than the light contact used for acupuncture holding points

- Pressure is generally held for three to ten seconds or one minute depending upon the severity of the condition

- Chronic and acute conditions usually require repeated applications of pressure to effect an improvement; however, under certain circumstances immediate results are noted after one application

- Shiatsu treatment need not be a painful experience, although occasional discomfort is sometimes inevitable

- Shiatsu evolved from ancient Chinese techniques of massage and manipulation in the early part of this century

- Each point along a meridian corresponds to and helps effect a change in a particular organ or part of the body

- Shiatsu encourages the body's natural healing mechanism to function optimally

- Shiatsu is administered slowly, quietly and with great compassion

d) REFLEXOLOGY *Hand & Foot*

- The body is divided into ten different zones which extend into the feet and the hands *See page 44*

- Each area of the foot corresponds to a specific organ or part of the body

- Nerves that pass through the body's organs and muscles terminate in the hands and feet

- Applying pressure to a particular area of the foot or hand stimulates the flow of energy, blood, nutrients and nerve impulses to its corresponding zone of the body

- Crystalline deposits of uric acid and calcium that form at the nerve endings prevent the nerve from functioning at its peak efficiency

- Pressure applied to the reflex points disintegrates crystalline deposits on the nerve endings. it also affects the entire nerve as well as those muscles and organs it innervates

- Once crushed, crystalline deposits can be re-absorbed into the bloodstream and excreted in the urine

- Reflexology stimulates the body's own natural healing mechanism

- A firm pressure is required, but the object is NOT to inflict pain

- Two or three applications of pressure daily are required to effect a change in a condition

- There are many different schools of reflexology, each with its own interpretation of where the reflex points are located

- All schools agree, however, that the precise locations of the nerve endings vary slightly in each individual

- The following charts take into consideration many different schools, plus some of the author's own discoveries *See page 43 and 67*

HAND REFLEXOLOGY

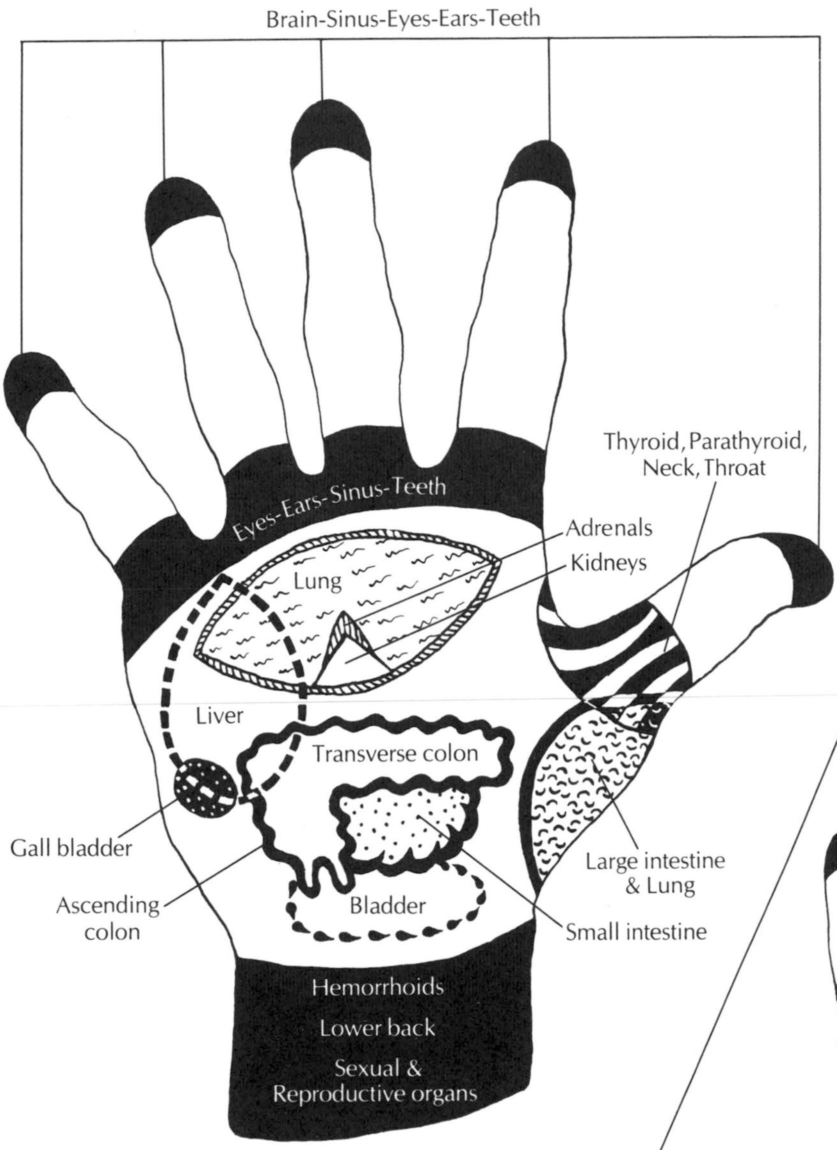

Brain-Sinus-Eyes-Ears-Teeth

Eyes-Ears-Sinus-Teeth

Thyroid, Parathyroid, Neck, Throat

Adrenals

Kidneys

Lung

Liver

Transverse colon

Gall bladder

Ascending colon

Bladder

Large intestine & Lung

Small intestine

Hemorrhoids

Lower back

Sexual & Reproductive organs

RIGHT

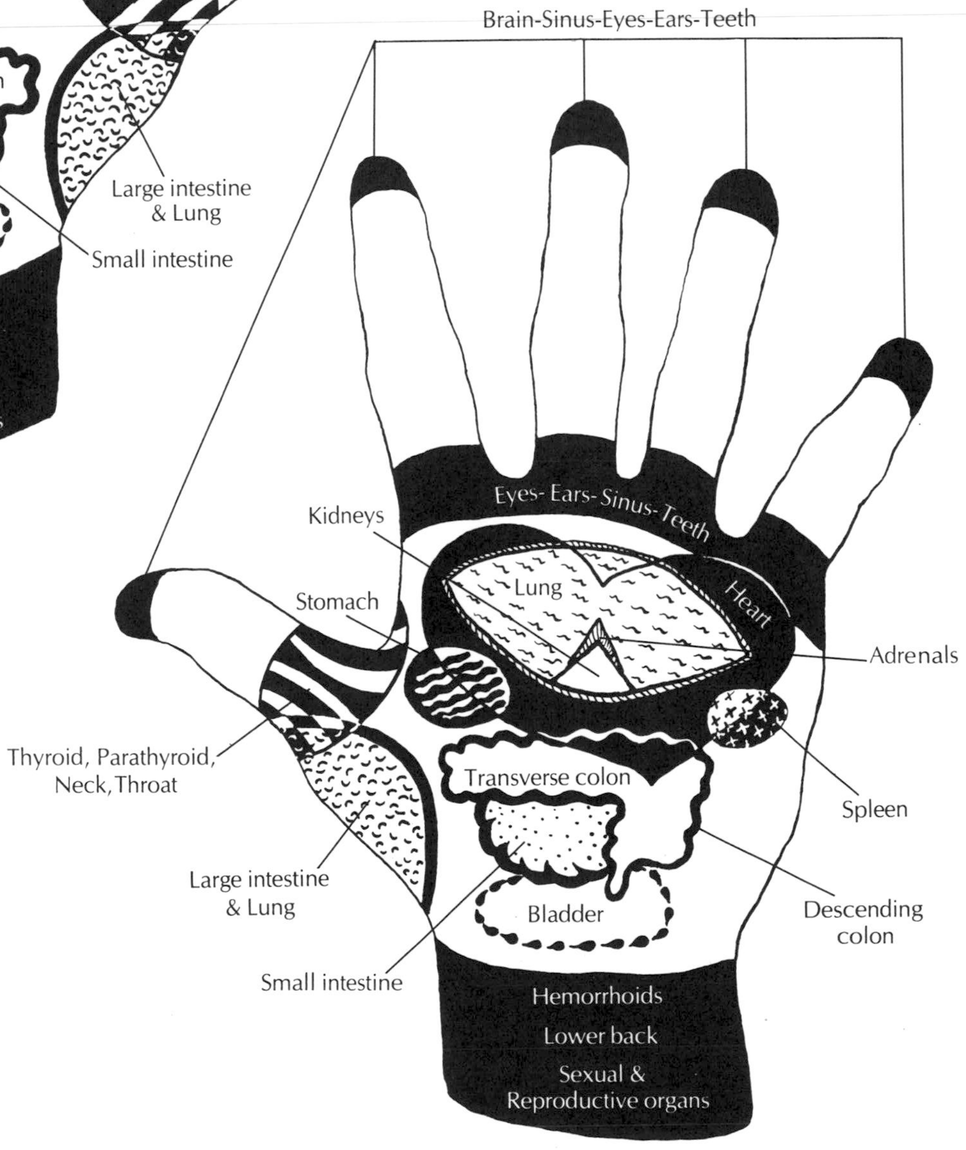

Brain-Sinus-Eyes-Ears-Teeth

Eyes-Ears-Sinus-Teeth

Heart

Kidneys

Stomach

Lung

Adrenals

Spleen

Thyroid, Parathyroid, Neck, Throat

Transverse colon

Large intestine & Lung

Bladder

Descending colon

Small intestine

Hemorrhoids

Lower back

Sexual & Reproductive organs

LEFT

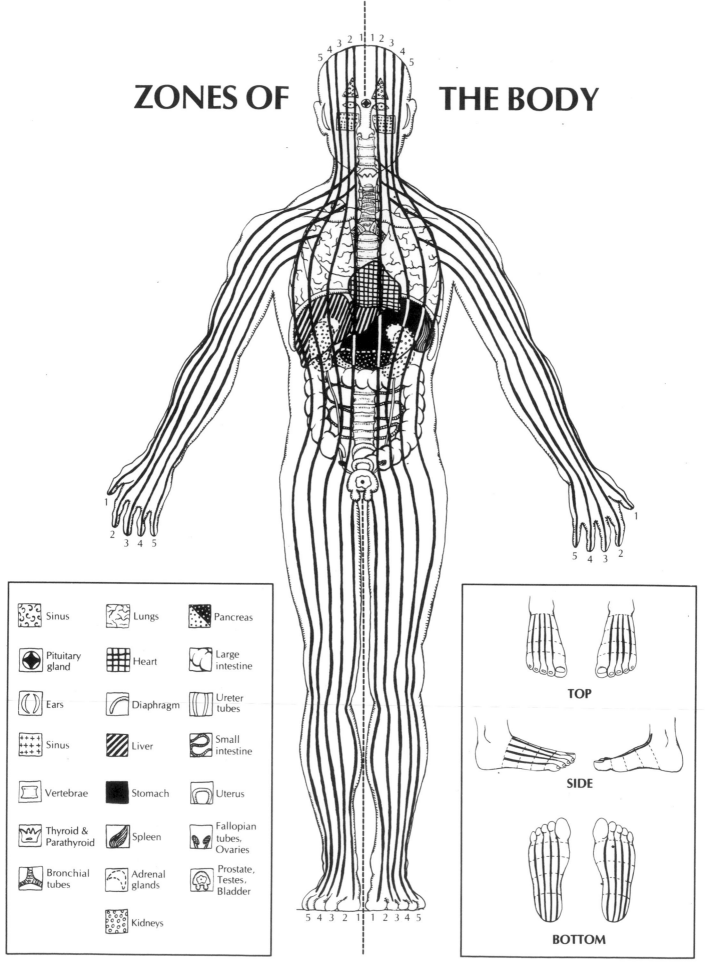

ZONES OF THE BODY

Sinus	Lungs	Pancreas
Pituitary gland	Heart	Large intestine
Ears	Diaphragm	Ureter tubes
Sinus	Liver	Small intestine
Vertebrae	Stomach	Uterus
Thyroid & Parathyroid	Spleen	Fallopian tubes, Ovaries
Bronchial tubes	Adrenal glands	Prostate, Testes, Bladder
Kidneys		

TOP

SIDE

BOTTOM

e) TOUCH FOR HEALTH

Touch for Health utilizes the techniques of Applied Kinesiology to encourage the body's natural healing mechanism. Applied Kinesiology has derived some of its methods from Oriental Medicine. Some of the methods used to achieve results are:

1) *Muscle Testing*

2) *Neuro-vascular Holding Points*

3) *Neuro-lymphatic Massage Points*

4) *Meridian Tracing*

1) MUSCLE TESTING

- Applied Kinesiology is a science that has proven each muscle to be affected by the function of a particular organ(s)

- Muscle testing is the method used to determine if a muscle is strong or weak

- Muscle testing indicates the ability or inability of a muscle and its associated organ to function at peak energy efficiency

- Applied Kinesiology utilizes neuro-vascular holding points, neuro-lymphatic massage, meridian therapy, origin and insertion massage (simultaneously massaging the origin and insertion of a muscle), exercise and other methods to restore the proper function to the muscle and its related organ

- Applied Kinesiology is used extensively by chiropractors and the layperson's adaptation of it is taught by certified Touch for Health instructors

2) NEURO-VASCULAR HOLDING POINTS

- Neuro-vascular holding points or receptors were discovered in the 1930's by Dr. Terence Bennett

- George Goodheart, D.C., revealed the relationship between the neuro-vascular holding points and the musculoskeletal system

The neuro-vascular receptors, when blocked, will prevent the occurrence of the lactic acid response, which occurs naturally each time a muscle contracts

- Connect with the neuro-vascular holding points by applying a light finger-pad contact

- Feel for a light pulse not directly related to the heartbeat. If the pulse is difficult to locate, gently stretch the skin and the pulse will become noticeable

- This pulsation is thought to be a result of the capillary beds' microscopic throbbing

- Hold the receptors until the pulses become synchronized. This usually occurs within twenty seconds, although five, ten or more minutes may be necessary

- Neuro-vascular holding points are believed to improve the capillary circulation of blood to the muscle and its related organ

- Most of the neuro-vascular holding points are situated on the skull *See pages 148 & 149*

3) NEURO-LYMPHATIC MASSAGE POINTS

- Dr. Frank Chapman was the first to discover neuro-lymphatic massage points or receptors

- George Goodheart, D.C., systematically correlated each neuro-lymphatic receptor to one or more muscles

- When a neuro-lymphatic receptor is blocked, its correspondent muscles are unable to function normally

- Massage the neuro-lymphatics by applying a medium-firm pressure with your thumbs or fingers

- Those neuro-lymphatics that are tender are most in need of massage

- Use a clockwise massaging motion. If the tenderness does not disappear within fifteen to thirty seconds, switch to a counter-clockwise massaging motion

SCHEMATIC
THE LYMPHATIC DRAINAGE SYSTEM

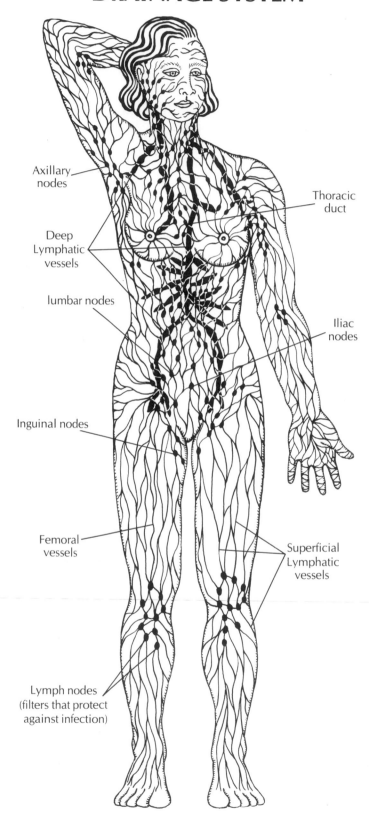

Axillary nodes

Deep Lymphatic vessels

lumbar nodes

Inguinal nodes

Femoral vessels

Lymph nodes (filters that protect against infection)

Thoracic duct

Iliac nodes

Superficial Lymphatic vessels

ANTERIOR

Lymph vessels return excess tissue fluid and cellular waste products to the blood stream.

NEURO-LYMPHATIC MASSAGE POINTS

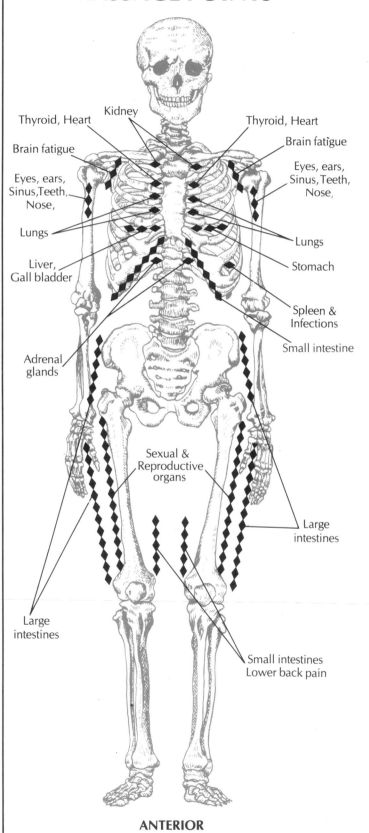

Thyroid, Heart

Kidney

Brain fatigue

Eyes, ears, Sinus,Teeth, Nose,

Lungs

Liver, Gall bladder

Adrenal glands

Large intestines

Thyroid, Heart

Brain fatigue

Eyes, ears, Sinus,Teeth, Nose,

Lungs

Stomach

Spleen & Infections

Small intestine

Sexual & Reproductive organs

Large intestines

Small intestines Lower back pain

ANTERIOR

- The neuro-lymphatics generally become less tender as you massage them, for release of the backed-up lymphatic system is being achieved

- Most of the neuro-lymphatics are located on the torso (front and back), although some are located on the legs and arms

- If the neuro-lymphatic tenderness still exists after fifteen or thirty seconds of first clockwise and then counter-clockwise massaging, the muscle and organ associated with the particular neuro-lymphatic will require many more applications over a period of time in order for the blockage to be released

- The neuro-lymphatic massage points or receptors flush the body's lymph system.

- When a body is overloaded with toxins, the lymphatic receptors become tender or painful to the touch, and act as an alarm system

- Some of the neuro-lymphatic massage points correspond to the location of the lymph glands or nodules; however, many do not directly relate in a physical sense

- The lymph is also responsible for the transport of fats, hormones and proteins as well as for the production of antibodies

4) MERIDIAN TRACING

- Lightly trace or follow the line or course of a meridian several times from its origin to its termination

- If tracing a meridian from its origin to its point of termination makes the receiver feel uneasy, try reversing the flow of the meridian several times or alternating its flow from origin to termination and then from termination to origin a few times. This is known as flushing a meridian. Complete the procedure by tracing the meridian several times in the correct direction. This procedure will often correct the flow of a meridian that is reversed *Refer to pages 38 & 39 for the exact location of the meridians for tracing purposes.*

f) SWEDISH MASSAGE

- Swedish massage improves blood and lymph circulation

- It breaks down adhesions, reduces swelling and encourages wounds to heal

- It improves the flexibility of joints and increases their range of motion

- When using effleurage on the limbs, always begin at the extremity and continue upward toward the heart in order to return stagnant blood back to the heart for recirculation

- Swedish massage uses more vigorous and stimulating techniques than Shiatsu

- There are five basic massage techniques:

  1) Effleurage—a long stroking motion, deep or superficial, in the direction of the heart, to improve circulation and lymph flow throughout the body as well as to improve nutrition and functioning of muscles

  2) Petrissage—the kneading, picking up, squeezing and rolling of the muscles to stimulate the deep blood and lymph vessels and to strengthen the muscles

  3) Friction—a penetrating circular movement, applied primarily to the joints, to effect destruction of adhesions

  4) Vibration— of the forearm, hand and fingers to stimulate the nervous system

  5) Tapotment—a chopping, slapping, hacking, beating, cupping motion, implemented with the hands open or closed, to stimulate the muscles — Tapotment can also either sedate or stimulate the nerves, depending upon the duration and intensity of its application

- Swedish massage does not, for the most part, claim to affect or assist directly the functioning of internal organs. Nor does it concern itself with the movement of energy or the meridian system and its pressure points

THE BLOOD CIRCULATORY SYSTEM
SCHEMATIC

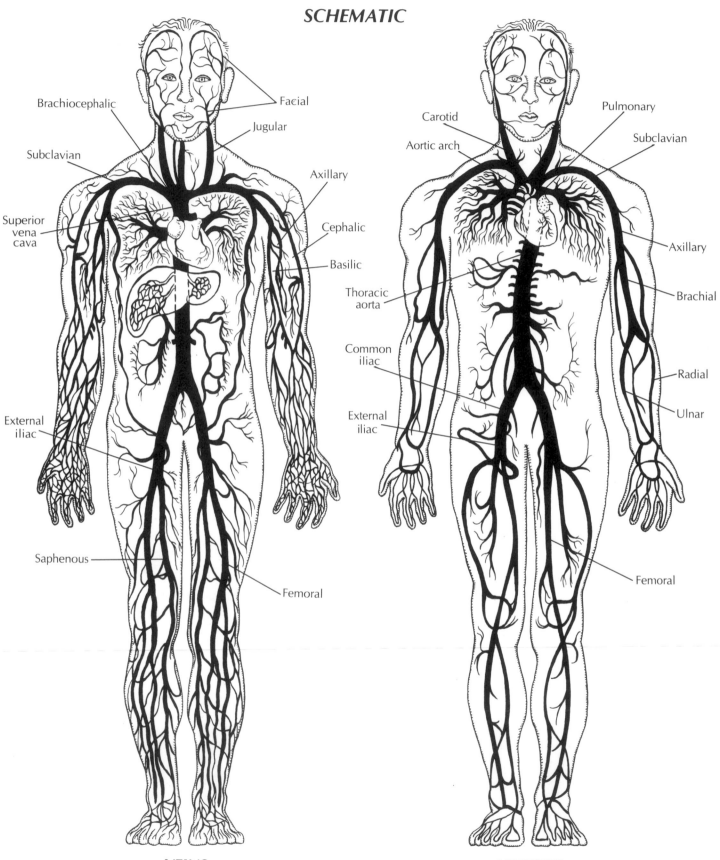

Brachiocephalic

Facial

Jugular

Subclavian

Axillary

Superior vena cava

Cephalic

Basilic

External iliac

Saphenous

Femoral

Carotid

Pulmonary

Aortic arch

Subclavian

Axillary

Thoracic aorta

Brachial

Common iliac

External iliac

Radial

Ulnar

Femoral

VEINS

Veins transport deoxygenated blood to the heart and lungs for recirculation.

ARTERIES

Arteries transport oxygenated blood away from the heart to all parts of the body.

6)BASIC SKELETAL & MUSCULAR ANATOMY

- Bones fall into four categories: long, short, flat and irregular

- All bones have a porous inner portion and an outer covering of hard, compact bone

- Bones provide support and protection as well as making movement possible in coordination with the muscular system

- Bones are found in pairs, one on each side of the body

- Bones store calcium and form red blood cells

- Nutrient rich blood and lymph fluids move into and out of bone tissue

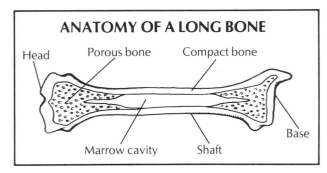

ANATOMY OF A LONG BONE

Head
Porous bone
Compact bone
Marrow cavity
Shaft
Base

The following skeletal charts will give you a good sense of the bony structure or foundation that provides places of attachment for all the muscles, so that you will not harm the receiver while implementing pressure points. Have someone lie down on the floor. Try to visualize where the bones are located in the person's body. If you cannot quite determine a bone's location, feel for it while making frequent visual checks to the following charts.

- Muscles consist of fibers or cells, which, if contracted, pull bones and effect movement of the body

- Muscles are found in pairs, one on each side of the body

- All muscles have two ends, an origin and an insertion, which attach or connect to bones, ligaments or cartilage

- The origin of a muscle is usually closer to the center of your body

- The belly of a muscle is the fullest or broadest part of a muscle

- Massaging the origin and insertion of a muscle in unison helps to strengthen that muscle

- You can relax a muscle by feathering, by a light gliding motion or by a medium-pressure pulling motion. When implementing any of these techniques, work from the belly of the muscle toward the origin and insertion in order to relieve muscle cramps or spasms

- The same feathering and pulling motions, when utilized from the origin and insertion toward the belly of the muscle, will strengthen a weak muscle

- Muscles store physical and emotional trauma which form a knot or hard spot. Such traumatized areas are usually swollen to some degree and hotter than healthy, normal tissue and are also known as adhesions or energy blockages

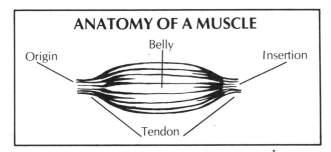

ANATOMY OF A MUSCLE

Origin
Belly
Insertion
Tendon

The following muscle charts must be reviewed before beginning your first massage. It is helpful to the beginner to have an understanding and mental image of the major muscles of the body. Remember, you are not massaging or applying pressure to the skin, but to the muscles and the core of the body. A deep, penetrating massage or pressure need not be painful. An understanding of the muscular system will allow you to handle the body skillfully and with great compassion.

THE SKELETAL SYSTEM

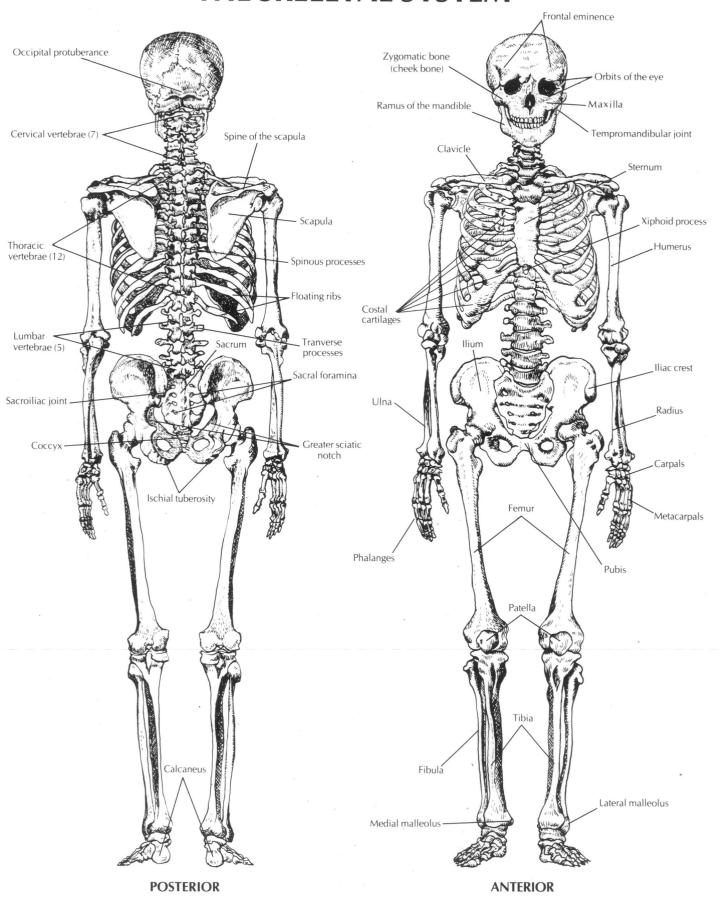

Occipital protuberance

Cervical vertebrae (7)

Spine of the scapula

Scapula

Thoracic vertebrae (12)

Spinous processes

Floating ribs

Lumbar vertebrae (5)

Sacrum

Tranverse processes

Sacral foramina

Sacroiliac joint

Coccyx

Greater sciatic notch

Ischial tuberosity

Calcaneus

POSTERIOR

Frontal eminence

Zygomatic bone (cheek bone)

Orbits of the eye

Ramus of the mandible

Maxilla

Tempromandibular joint

Clavicle

Sternum

Xiphoid process

Humerus

Costal cartilages

Ilium

Iliac crest

Ulna

Radius

Carpals

Metacarpals

Phalanges

Femur

Pubis

Patella

Tibia

Fibula

Lateral malleolus

Medial malleolus

ANTERIOR

50

THE MUSCULAR SYSTEM

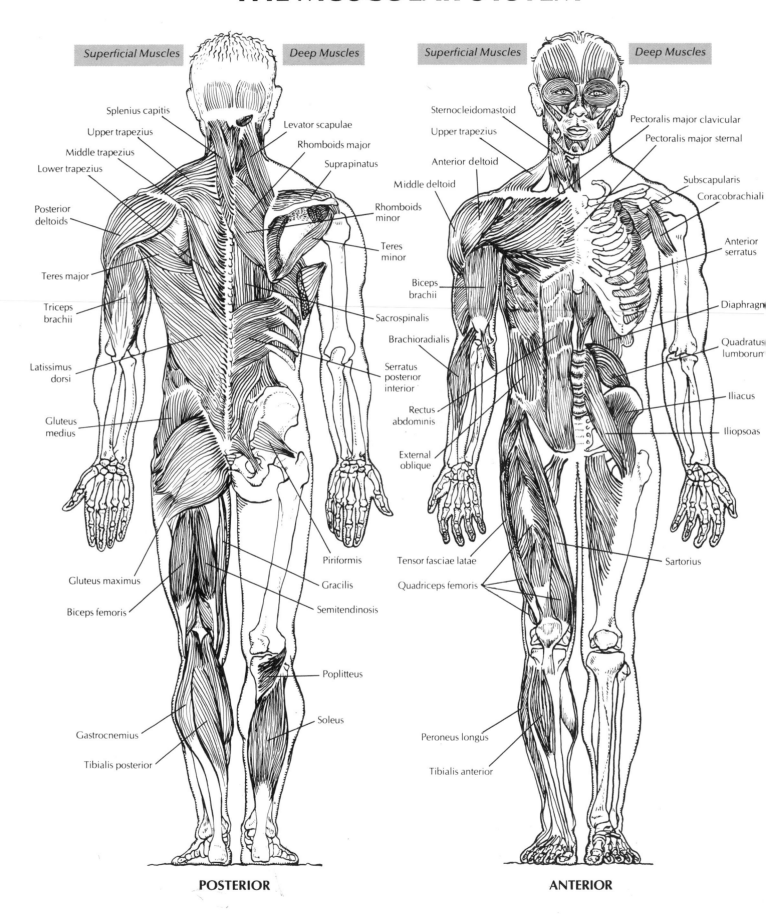

Superficial Muscles   Deep Muscles

Splenius capitis
Upper trapezius
Middle trapezius
Lower trapezius

Posterior deltoids

Teres major

Triceps brachii

Latissimus dorsi

Gluteus medius

Gluteus maximus

Biceps femoris

Gastrocnemius

Tibialis posterior

Levator scapulae
Rhomboids major
Suprapinatus
Rhomboids minor
Teres minor

Sacrospinalis

Serratus posterior interior

Piriformis
Gracilis
Semitendinosis

Poplitteus

Soleus

POSTERIOR

Superficial Muscles   Deep Muscles

Sternocleidomastoid
Upper trapezius
Anterior deltoid
Middle deltoid

Biceps brachii

Brachioradialis

Rectus abdominis

External oblique

Pectoralis major clavicular
Pectoralis major sternal
Subscapularis
Coracobrachiali
Anterior serratus
Diaphragm
Quadratus lumborun
Iliacus
Iliopsoas

Tensor fasciae latae
Quadriceps femoris

Peroneus longus
Tibialis anterior

Sartorius

ANTERIOR

51

CHAPTER IV

How to Give A Complete 60-Minute Body Massage

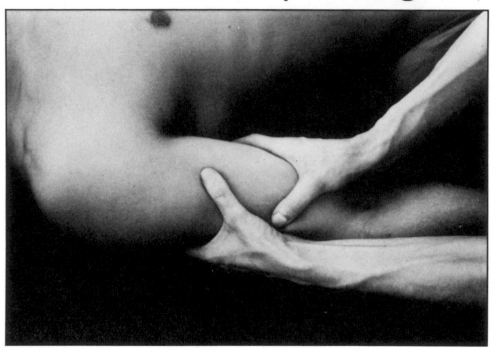

INTRODUCTION

The Complete 60-Minute Body Massage is intended for use by couples or friends who would like to exchange massages on a regular weekly basis. Partners should read this section together and practice each technique prior to the first massage, not only to gain knowledge of each of the procedures but also to share the actual physical experience of each technique. Consequently, the receiver will relax more easily and the doer will feel more self-confident. The massage, in turn, will be a more rewarding exchange. This introduction is written primarily for the doer, although some mention is made of the receiver's responsibility.

Responsibility and commitment to the massage are essential components of its success. Both the doer and the receiver must be prepared to fulfill their responsibilities in order to assure a pleasurable exchange.

As the receiver, you must make every effort to relax. You should breathe slowly and take deeper breaths when a pressure point is tender or painful. Your deep inhalation will alert the doer to reduce the force of the pressure being applied. Words are usually unnecessary, but if the deep breathing method fails to alert the doer to your discomfort, verbally express your malaise and request that less pressure be applied. Don't hide the pain you feel. Avoid talking as much as possible. Speak only when it is absolutely necessary, and let the magic of massage flow from the doer's hands into your body. Keep your eyes closed. Allow your mind to free-associate. Don't focus on your thoughts, but simply let them pass or wander through your mind. As the receiver, it is your responsibility NOT to help the doer by lifting your arms, legs or head. Since the doer is usually strong enough to lift your appendages, your help is unnecessary. Finally, if you, as the receiver, find yourself falling asleep, don't fight it, surrender completely and let go.

It is the doer's responsibility to be calm, compassionate and in control, for otherwise the receiver will not feel secure enough to let go. Perform techniques slowly. Quick or vigorous massaging is not conducive to the calm you wish to achieve and prevents the receiver's body from achieving deep relaxation. Whenever you utilize kneading techniques, perform them slowly without the use of oils.

Improved blood and lymphatic circulation can also be effected through slowly executed massage and pressure techniques. Your aim is to sedate, not stimulate, the receiver. As life offers more than enough stimulation, massage, in my opinion, should be sedating in order to provide maximum benefits. Once the body has been successfully relaxed, so that energy blockages as well as muscle tension can be released, the lymph and blood circulation will automatically improve. Sedation of the receiver's mind and body is the most effective way to release stored tension on both the emotional and physical levels.

It is also the doer's responsibility to remind the receiver to breathe. The reminder can be verbal, or you can exaggerate your inhaling and exhaling until the receiver gets the message. Most people hold their breath without knowing it. If you allow the receiver to do so frequently throughout a massage, the results will be less releasing and less relaxing.

Avoid losing contact with the receiver's body whenever you change techniques or switch positions. Always keep one hand or some part of your body in contact with the receiver's body. If you do not, the receiver will usually experience a mild shock due to the unexpected withdrawal. The eyes will suddenly open and the receiver will often sit up with a start and wonder if something is wrong. When it is absolutely necessary that you remove yourself entirely from the receiver's body, your departure and your return to contact must be very gradual, so that the receiver doesn't experience a feeling of separation. Generally, it is far simpler to remain in constant contact with the receiver's body.

Occasionally the receiver may say, "Oh, that feels good!" or "Could you do more of that technique?" You, as the doer should always acknowledge such comments. Tell the receiver that you will remain with the technique a little longer than usual and that you will return to it later during the massage. A receiver's compliment to you on a particular technique usually indicates the fulfillment of a great physical or emotional need. Often the receiver will sigh deeply rather than speak. A deep sigh also signals your duty to spend a little more time on the technique. Do not deny the receiver. The extra attention you give to a particular need communicates your understanding, your sensitivity and your willingness to help the receiver. It will also significantly increase the benefits of the particular technique.

There are three basic degrees of pressure: light, medium and heavy. No set standard exists for any of these three degrees, as each person is capable of enjoying and tolerating different amounts of pressure and pain. Learn your receiver's tolerance level and observe the face for indications of pain or pleasure. Remember, too, that firm pressure is not always applied with the same amount of force, even when massaging the same receiver. For example, firm pressure applied to the eyes will obviously differ in force from firm pressure applied to the arms or legs. The part of the body being massaged or receiving pressure determines how much force you apply. It is extremely difficult to describe the application of pressure without becoming slightly esoteric. The application of heavy pressure without causing the receiver pain is esssential to the successful practice of massage. Even some professional massage therapists do not know how to apply pressure correctly, so don't be to discouraged if you fail to grasp the method of application immediately.

Pressure applied incorrectly results in a brutal, insensitive massage. The pressure you apply must be the end-result of a magical force hidden deep within you and rising up from your hara, then following down your arms and into the receiver's body. Hara, remember, is the Japanese word for the center of the energy of your body and is located approximately one-and-a-half inches below your navel. Here resides the strength and the sensitivity needed to accomplish a successful, compassionate and magical massage.

The Japanese believe that when you function from the hara, you can achieve what would normally be difficult or impossible. Hara, in Western terms, can most easily be described as functioning from your gut or relying on your instincts. You've heard of "gut reaction." Gut reactions are almost always correct or accurate. For example, imagine you are with someone when they receive shocking news over the telephone. Your gut reaction or instincts tell you to hold or console the person. Or imagine you are walking down the street and coming toward you is someone who looks like trouble. Chances are, your instincts will tell you to cross the street to avoid the trouble. By the same token, if you apply pressure or massage from your hara, you will instinctively know how much pressure to apply. Do not consciously try to determine how much pressure to apply. Let your instincts or gut reaction be your guide. Remember, don't use muscle power. Pain is not your objective. Use hara or gut force. Excellent results can be achieved with less pressure and a minimum of pain.

There are several different types of pain. It is important to be aware of the type with which you are dealing as you massage. Always apply pressure slowly, and take the time to notice the receiver's reaction in order to reduce the possibility of inflicting pain.

1) "Tender" means that the pressure applied hurts a little, but not enough to worry about

2) "Good pain" hurts, but the receiver knows or can feel that the pressure is helping and therefore, the pain is worth tolerating

3) "Bad pain" is usually the result of too much pressure, of a slip of the hand or thumb, or of pressure beyond the receiver's tolerance threshold

Whenever you apply pressure that causes pain, the doer should be sure to "make nice" afterwards. Making nice indicates to the receiver that you are aware of the discomfort. It is also a perfect way to say, "I'm sorry." Make nice by giving a few light circular massages to the painful area or by gently holding the spot with your thumb, fingers or entire hand.

It is important to apply pressure slowly so that you can determine the shape of the bony structures under the skin. When you're certain of the form the bone assumes beneath a particular pressure point, you are less likely to slip and harm the receiver. When applying pressure to the limbs, each application should slightly "roll" or move the limb. If it doesn't, chances are that you are applying too much force behind your pressure or that the receiver is tense. Your aim is not to nail the limb to the floor. Again, remember to draw upon the force within your hara.

If the receiver has a diagnosed condition for the points you are utilizing, repeat the technique to increase the benefits. For example, by applying repeated pressure to the points that correspond to the liver, gall bladder, stomach, heart, spleen, lungs, eyes or ears, you can encourage the body's natural healing mechanism to take over and help to correct the condition.

Diseases or illnesses are either acute or chronic. Acute illnesses or conditions occur suddenly, and the symptoms are usually quite severe. Chronic illnesses have a long duration, sometimes months and often years, and are conditions that recur frequently. Whether chronic or acute, most illnesses respond well to frequently repeated applications of pressure or massage. The more frequently the organs' corresponding points are contacted, the greater the results. Contacting these points several times daily will, over a period of time, speed the recovery of both acute and chronic conditions.

Don't get discouraged. Keep at it. As most conditions take years to evolve, you can't expect to improve or cure them overnight. Rarely will you notice immediate results. Weeks or months are usually needed in order to effect a significantly noticeable difference. Some improvement is, however, usually apparent after one or two weeks of frequent daily applications. Patience will reward you.

The Complete 60-Minute Body Massage is a synthesis of Acupuncture pressure points, Shiatsu, Touch for Health, Foot Reflexology, Swedish Massage and original techniques. The meridians, acupuncture points, neuro-lymphatic drainage points, reflex points and Swedish techniques illustrated in this chapter were briefly discussed in Chapter III, Section 5.

The muscles and bones mentioned in this section are diagrammed in Chapter III, Section 6. Review the drawings before attempting to give your first massage. This basic anatomical information is essential to your success.

This section of *The Magic of Massage* occasionally mentions a relationship between a particular organ and muscle. Applied Kinesiology, discussed in Section 5e of Chapter III, has proven that specific muscles relate to particular organs. Whenever the text states that a particular muscle is related to a specific organ, the information has been derived from the science of Applied Chiropractic Kinesiological Diagnosis and Technique.

Feathering, utilized only once, in Technique #30 for Feathering the Spine, can also be used as a farewell to the part of the body you have been massaging and as a greeting to the part of the body you are about to massage. Feathering is done with the finger tips. Your aim is to create the sensation of a feather lightly gliding over the receiver's body. Maintain a very light contact with your finger tips while gliding them over the skin. Feathering can be done in any direction. Its light, gliding motion signals the brain to relax the area being feathered and thereby prepares it for massage or suggests a farewell. Feathering can be utilized before and after many of the techniques discussed in The Complete 60-Minute Body Massage. This feather in the margin or between techniques indicates an appropriate time to feather. The use of feathering is optional and is not included in the total time calculations. It is, however, a delightful addition to any massage.

The Complete 60-Minute Body Massage is presented in the following format:

NAME OF THE TECHNIQUE

Purpose: Why you do the technique and what organs, muscles or part of the body is affected.
Positioning: What position is most practical to assume. If this position is not comfortable for your particular body type, improvise until you find one that is.
Procedure: How to execute the technique, along with important tips to remember while implementing it.
Repetition: How many times the technique should be repeated during the massage.
Time: Approximately how much time is required to complete the technique. The time allotted cannot be very exacting, because each individual will require repetition of the techniques for the particular conditions that are troublesome to them. Obviously, someone who is very ill or rundown will require more repetitions than someone who is in reasonably good health.

Remember that in the magic of massage, fifty percent of the success is determined by the quality of your touch and fifty percent by your desire to help. Technique and know-how are important, but only as vehicles for your touch and your desire to help.

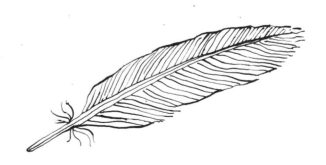

THE BACK

It is advisable to begin a massage with the back because many people experience a stiffening of the neck when lying in a prone position. The receiver must, after all, lie prone with the head turned to one side for the ten or fifteen minutes required by the doer to massage and apply pressure to the back. When you end a massage with the back, the receiver will often sit up, rotate the neck and try to massage it. Of course, the doer can, at this point, massage away the stiffness in the receiver's shoulders and tension in the neck, but it is psychologically unwise to conclude a session in this manner. Indeed, it's ridiculous to ruin one hour of wonderful manipulation by leaving the receiver with a pain in the neck. Therefore, unless you are sure the receiver will not develop a stiff neck, begin the massage with the back and follow the sequence of techniques listed below. Use slow, calm massaging motions and cautious, but firm applications of pressure to specific points.

All techniques should be executed quietly, slowly and with great compassion. There are two very important rules that must be remembered. One is NEVER to apply pressure directly over the spinous processes. The other is NEVER to apply

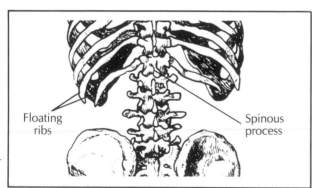

Floating ribs

Spinous process

too much open-handed pressure to the lower back, for there are no ribs in the lower back to absorb such pressure. Also, it is important that heavy pressure NOT be applied over the last two floating ribs as they can break quite easily.

For the sake of clarity some of the photographs do not show a pillow under the receiver's legs.

1) THE FIRST TOUCH

Purpose: The First Touch is a subtle way of letting the receiver know you are ready to begin. Words are unnecessary.

Positioning: Sit, Japanese style, parallel to the receiver between the body and the arm.

Procedure: The First Touch is executed with the side of your leg, not with your hands. Position yourself next to the receiver, but do not make contact at this time. The side of your body should be approximately 1-1½ inches from the receiver's body. Remain perfectly still for 10-15 seconds. Try to release everyday thoughts from your mind. To aid you, take a few breaths. When you are ready to begin, gently shift your body weight until your leg comes in contact with the side of the receiver's body. You have now completed the First Touch.

Repetition: Repetition of this technique is necessary only if you are interrupted and must start again.

Time: Allow 15 seconds to relax prior to making your first touch. When both you and the receiver are relaxed and ready to begin, allow your leg to make contact. You will learn to sense when the time is right. Allow a few seconds of leg contact before proceeding to the next technique. Total time: 20 seconds.

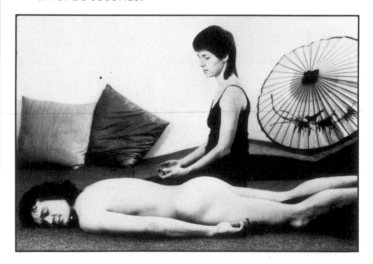

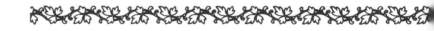

2) THE LAYING-ON OF HANDS

Purpose: The initial hand contact is of utmost importance. If compassion, sensitivity and confidence are expressed in the doer's hand, they will establish the proper tone and mood for the rest of the massage. Your hands must touch the receiver with authority and a gentle strength so that the receiver feels your hands are safe hands. Your initial contact should immediately secure the receiver's trust and submission in order for you to perform your part of the massage, which is GIVING. You cannot effectively give unless the receiver is willing to receive. The receiver must allow the doer to penetrate into the very essence of her/his being.

Positioning: Sit parallel to the receiver, Japanese style.

Procedure: Keep your leg in contact with the receiver's body as you proceed, very slowly and quietly, to *gently* lay one hand on the sacrum and then to lay the other directly over the spine between the scapulae (shoulder blades). Let your hands settle into the receiver's back the way butter melts into a pancake. When your hands are at full rest, your entire body should be relaxed. Maintain this contact for approximately 30 seconds. Be sure your wrists and hands are supple and relaxed, as tense hands will communicate tension to the receiver. Synchronize your breathing with the receiver's by audibly inhaling and ex-

haling at the receiver's rate at least five times. Then indicate to the receiver that you want to slow down the breathing rate by taking loud, deep, slow breaths. In a few seconds the receiver will sense your desire to relax and be one, and will usually sigh very deeply to indicate submission and readiness. Indeed, this deep sigh signifies the receiver is "in the now" of the massage, and you can proceed to the next technique, Spine Tracing.

Repetition: Repeat this technique only if you have been disturbed and must begin again.

Time: The entire technique will usually be accomplished in 60 seconds.

3) SPINE TRACING

Purpose: Spine Tracing relaxes the receiver and helps to eliminate superficial spinal tension. Spine Tracing also affords an excellent opportunity for the doer to make mental notes of hard, dry, puffy, flaky, scaly, hot or cold spots along the spine. These are the outward manifestations of inner disturbances. You will need to pay more attention to these spots when you begin Vertebrae Technique #6.

Positioning: Sit, Japanese style, as in Techniques #1 and #2.

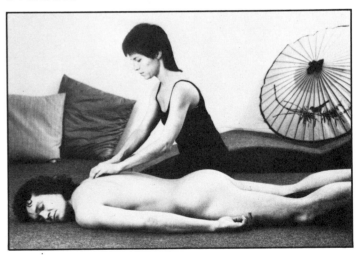

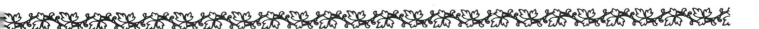

Procedure: Place three fingers on either side of the spine. Begin as close to the base of the skull as possible, and *very slowly,* with a medium pressure, pull your fingers all the way down either side of the spine. Continue over the sacrum and end at the tip of the coccyx. Remember to make mental notes of unusual muscle tension, skin textures or temperature changes of the skin along the spine.

Repetition: Repeat Spine Tracing two or three times.

Time: 40 seconds.

4) ROCKING THE BACK

Purpose: This technique serves further to loosen and relax the muscles of the back, as well as to prepare it for the heavy thumb pressure of Vertebrae Technique #5. It also feels very good.

Positioning: Sit, Japanese style, with your body perpendicular to the receiver's spine. The actual rocking motion will be performed in a slightly raised position.

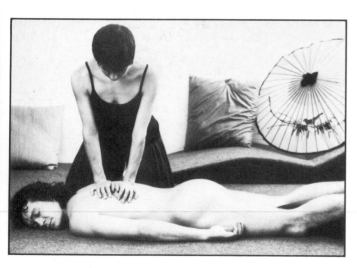

Procedure: Use the heels of your hands. Begin at the shoulders, one inch away from the spinal column. Holding your hands side by side, move them in unison back and forth in a rocking motion. As you proceed downward to the next area of the back, slightly overlap the area previously rocked in order to insure that no part of the back is neglected. Use your body weight to achieve the

rocking motion. *Do not use muscle power.* Rock all the way down to the sacrum. After you have completed one side, cross over the body and do the other side.

Repetition: Rock each area along the spine back and forth five times. Rock each side of the spine only once.

Time: 60 seconds.

5) DEEP BREATHING TECHNIQUE

Purpose: This technique helps the receiver release tension stored in the muscles of the back. It also relieves pressure on the nerves as they emerge from the spinal column.

Positioning: See Technique #6, Vertebrae Technique.

Procedure: Place your hands on either side of the spine near the neck. Ask the receiver to inhale. Then, as the receiver exhales, slowly allow your

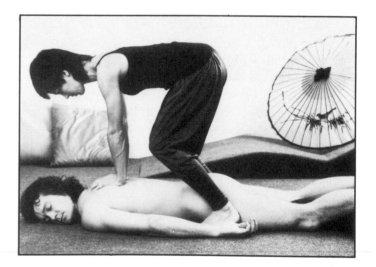

body weight to extend down your arms into your hands. Verbally encourage the receiver to exhale completely, for many people only partially exhale what they inhale. The pressure must be applied calmly so the receiver's back muscles don't tighten up in response to sudden pressure. Press when the receiver exhales as you continue down the spine to the coccyx.

Repetition: No repetition necessary.

Time: 30 seconds.

6) VERTEBRAE TECHNIQUE

Purpose: The Vertebrae Technique is executed in three phases.

PHASE	PURPOSE
1) Medium pressure, clockwise circular thumb massage.	Preparation for penetration by superficial relaxation of the back.
2) Firm penetrating pressure, executed with compassion, on either side of the spine. Use your thumbs.	Penetrating pressure releases tensions and triggers the body's natural healing mechanism.
3) Soothing, light, clockwise circular thumb massage.	"Making Nice." Alleviation of pain or discomfort caused by Phase 2:

Phase 3 of Vertebrae Technique is very important. It is essential to "make nice" because pain creates tension. By gently massaging the area affected, you encourage the receiver's body to release any pain or tension that has accumulated as a direct result of your firm thumb pressure in *Phase 2*. Remember, your aim is not to cause pain. You will, however, encounter areas that are tender or painful to the touch. Do not avoid these areas. Massage the sore spots. Be thorough, and be compassionate. Let your efforts be rewarded with the knowledge that the receiver's body will ultimately be experiencing less discomfort, improved energy and better blood circulation.

Positioning: There are three possible positions.

1) Straddle the receiver's body at the waist on your knees.

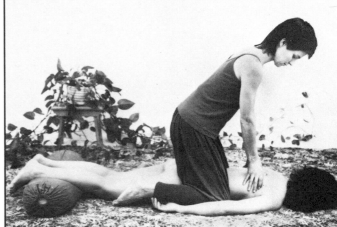

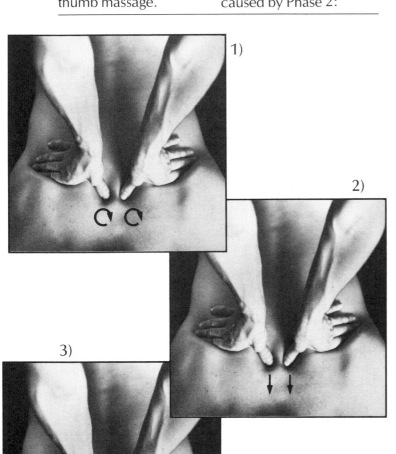

1)

2)

3)

59

2) Sit, Japanese style, at the receiver's side, parallel to the spine.

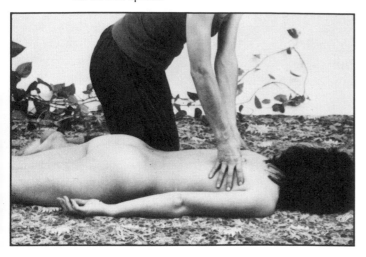

3) Stand, legs bent, straddling the receiver's body.

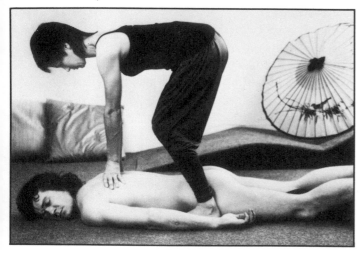

POSITION 1: is appropriate if the receiver is physically small enough for you to straddle. Do not sit or rest your body weight on the receiver.

POSITION 2: is used when the receiver is small enough for the doer to apply pressure evenly to both sides of the spinal column from one side of the body. As some people find Position 1 difficult to hold because their legs are spread apart, Position 2 is offered as an alternative. If you decide to use Position 2, be sure to apply equal pressure to both sides of the spinal column. Also, remember to keep your spine erect while you work. If you work in a slumped posture, you are very likely to strain your back muscles.

POSITION 3: is especially useful when the receiver is significantly larger than the doer. The extra height achieved in this raised position makes it easier for the doer to use body weight, rather than muscle power, to apply pressure. Position 3 also encourages equal distribution of body weight, because the doer is positioned directly over the receiver.

Procedure: Begin vertebrae massage and pressure on either side of and between the fifth and sixth thoracic vertebrae. See drawing.

There are two ways of locating the fifth and sixth thoracic vertebrae.

1) The lower tip of the scapula (shoulder blade) usually ends between the seventh and eighth intercostal space. Be sure the receiver's arms are stretched out at the side of the body, then count the spinous processes up from the base of the scapula to the fifth and sixth thoracic vertebrae.

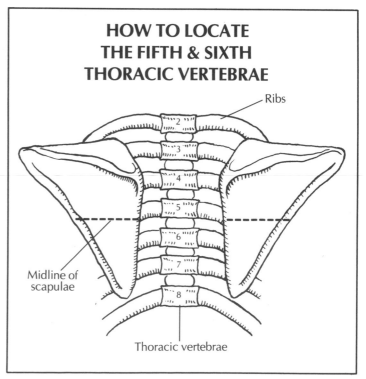

HOW TO LOCATE THE FIFTH & SIXTH THORACIC VERTEBRAE

Ribs

Midline of scapulae

Thoracic vertebrae

2) Eye-ball or approximate the location of the fifth and sixth thoracic by estimating the middle of the scapula. Midway between the top and bottom of the scapula is generally the location of the fifth and sixth thoracic vertebrae.

Once you have located the fifth and sixth thoracic vertebrae, begin implementing first *Phase 1*, then *Phase 2* and finally *Phase 3* on either side of and between each pair of the thoracic and lumbar vertebrae. There are twelve thoracic vertebrae, but for now you can ignore the first through the fifth, and there are five lumbar vertebrae. The lumbar vertebrae are located directly below the thoracic and terminate at the sacrum. Pressure must be applied perpendicularly to the plane of the body you are working. If the application of pressure is not perpendicular to the surface, the doer risks strained arms, sore thumbs or sudden back pain. Do not massage or apply pressure directly to the vertebral processes. This could prove painful or even damaging to the receiver. Reserve working on the upper thoracic vertebrae until you are seated at the receiver's head.

Repetition: PHASE 1: Use a medium pressure, clockwise circular thumb massage on either side of the spine between the vertebrae. Repeat rotations three to five times. If an area feels particularly tense, increase the number of rotations.

PHASE 2: Apply a firm penetrating pressure, executed with compassion, to either side of the spine between the transverse processes. The pressure is applied directly over the nerve as it emerges from the spinal column. Use your thumbs. If an area is particularly tense, release and repeat the pressure two or three times. Hold each application of pressure for 5 seconds.

PHASE 3: Use a light, soothing, clockwise circular thumb massaging motion. Repeat rotation three to five times, depending upon the intensity of the pain in that area when you were doing Phase 2.

Time: The entire mid and lower back will consume approximately five minutes of the massage. If the receiver is particularly tense, you will need to allot more time to complete this portion of the back.

7) SACRUM PRESSURE

Purpose: This technique relieves sacral tension and improves the flow of energy to the small intestines, bladder and sexual organs.

Positioning: There are three possible positions.

1) Sit parallel to the receiver's body.
2) Straddle the receiver's body on your knees.
3) Stand, legs bent, straddling the receiver.

Procedure: Locate the sacral foramina, the four holes on either side of the sacrum that transmit the sacral nerves and arteries. Once you have found these foramina, apply firm pressure to each of the depressions. Do both sides simultaneously.

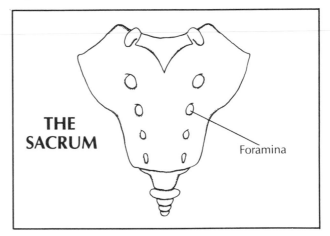

THE SACRUM

Foramina

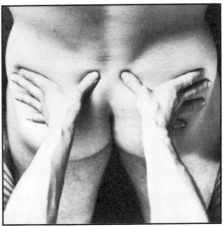

Repetition: No repetition is necessary, unless the receiver has a problem with either the small intestines, bladder or sexual organs.

Time: Hold the pressure over each of the foramina for 3-5 seconds. Total time: approximately 20 seconds.

8) BACK RELAXING & BROADENING STRETCH

Purpose: This technique suggests to the receiver's brain and back that you want the muscles of the back to broaden and relax. The stretch also feels very good.

Positioning: Same as #6, though Position 3 is most effective in this case, i.e. standing, legs bent, straddling the receiver's body.

Procedure: Begin by placing your thumbs on either side of the sacrum. Pull the thumbs out and away from the sacrum. Gently pulling the skin as

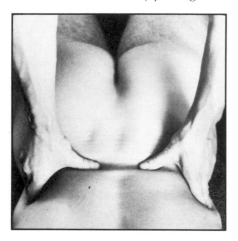

you move outward, slide the thumbs along the flesh and over the buttocks. Move up the sacrum one thumb space at a time, until you have covered the area entirely. Repeat the same technique, beginning on either side of and between the fourth and fifth lumbar vertebrae, and move up the back until you reach the neck.

Repetition: No repetition is necessary.

Time: Approximately 60 seconds.

9) WAIST & HIP LIFT

Purpose: This technique helps to trim the waistline. It also stimulates liver and gall bladder function.

Positioning: This technique is most efficiently done while straddling the receiver on your feet with your knees bent, but it can also be done while kneeling at the receiver's side.

Procedure: Slide your hands around and under

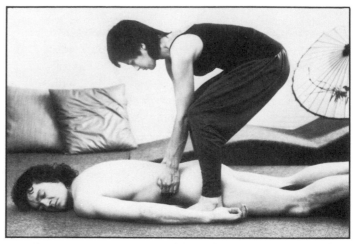

the receiver's waist. Holding the waist firmly, pull up with your hands. If the receiver is small-boned and not overweight, you may actually be able to lift the body slightly off the mat. It is not necessary to achieve this lift. It is only necessary to lift the flesh of the waist. If you can manage it easily, however, don't hesitate to lift the body up off the mat. Then, grasping the hip bones, lift the hips and buttocks off the mat.

Repetition: Lift the waist and hips twice.

Time: 30 seconds.

10) KNEADING OF THE BUTTOCKS

Purpose: Pressure and massage of the buttocks area is beneficial to the sciatic nerve, which is the largest nerve in the body. You are also massaging the gluteus maximus and gluteus medius muscles. Applied Kinesiology has proven that specific muscles correspond to particular organs. The gluteals correspond to the sexual and reproductive organs. The condition of these muscles can influence the general health and functioning of their related organs. For example, people who have weak or flabby gluteus muscles will often have ovary, uterus, womb or prostate problems. As these muscles often are flabby, they need massage to tone the loose flesh and improve the energy flow to the sexual and reproductive organs.

Positioning: Straddle the receiver's legs on your knees. Keep your spine in the correct alignment as your work.

Procedure : Two basic techniques accomplish the desired results.

1) With the heels of your hands begin a light to medium circular massaging motion. The buttocks is very often tender or painful, so work with great compassion. Massage the entire buttocks area twice to prepare adequately for your subsequent firm heel pressure.

2) Apply a slow, firm pressure with the heel of your hand to the entire buttocks area. Apply the pressure gradually so that you will know if the receiver is beginning to feel pain. Do not apply pressure if it causes too much pain. A little "good" pain helps to release the tension and/or blockage, but you don't need to torture the receiver. When your pressure begins to cause some discomfort, discontinue further penetration and hold pressure for 5 seconds. The area will become less painful as the seconds pass, and the tension or energy blockage will be relieved to some extent. Chronic sciatic conditions require more applications of pressure than acute conditions.

Repetition: Technique 1: Massage the entire buttocks area several times.

Technique 2: Slowly apply firm heel-of-the-hand pressure to five different locations on the buttocks. Hold pressure 5 seconds.

Time: Allow approximately 30 seconds for massaging and 25 seconds for the heel-of-the-hand technique.

BACKS OF THE LEGS

When massaging the backs of the legs, you will be applying pressure to the Bladder Meridian. Stimulation of this meridian will help the body to correct bladder conditons. Frequent urination, frequent desire with scanty emission and pain during urination are some of the conditions known to respond to Bladder Meridian pressure. If you have a bladder or urinary tract infection, pressure applied to this meridian will encourage the body's natural healing mechanism to work more quickly. The Bladder Meridian also affects the functioning of the kidney hormone system, as well as the autonomic nervous system of the urinary and reproductive organs.

11) THIGH BLADDER MERIDIAN PRESSURE

Purpose: This technique relaxes the back of the legs and affects the Bladder Meridian.
Positioning: Kneel between the receiver's legs.
Procedure: Use the heels of your hands. Begin to apply pressure below the gluteus maximus

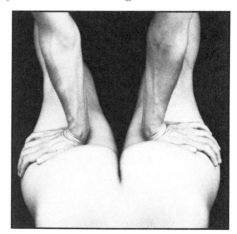

muscle, i.e. just below the buttocks. Do both legs at the same time, but alternate the firm pressure between the left heel and right heel of your hands as you move down the back of the leg to the crease of the knee. Hold each application of pressure 3-5 seconds.
Repetition: No repetition necessary.
Time: 20 seconds.

12) CREASE OF THE KNEE ACUPUNCTURE PRESSURE POINTS

Purpose: This technique effects a positive change in the Bladder Meridian and its related functions. It also releases tension stored in the knee.
Positioning: Kneel between the receiver's legs.
Procedure: Use your thumbs. Apply a firm, gentle and steady pressure to the center of the back of the crease of the knees. Keep your back aligned.

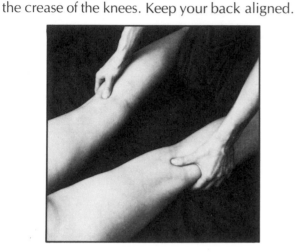

Repetition: Repeat the application of pressure three times and hold each for 3 seconds.
Time: Approximately 10 seconds.

13) LOWER BACK OF THE LEG BLADDER MERIDIAN PRESSURE

Purpose: Pressure here affects the Bladder Meridian and helps to relax the calf muscle. As the gastrocnemius, or calf muscle, correlates to the adrenal glands in Applied Kinesiology, you are also strengthening the functioning of the receiver's adrenal glands.
Positioning: Kneel between the receiver's legs.
Procedure: Use the heels of your hands to apply a slow, firm pressure down the center back of the calf muscle. The belly of the muscle, its widest part, cannot tolerate as much pressure as the rest of the leg. Be careful with your pressure here. Reduce it by half at the belly of the gastrocnemius.
Repetition: No repetition necessary.
Time: 20 seconds.

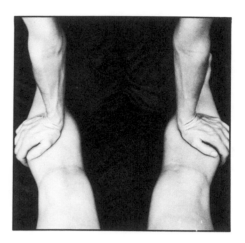

14) ACHILLES TENDON SQUEEZE

Purpose: Squeezing the Achilles tendon affects the prostate, uterus and rectum, as well as chronic sciatic nerve conditions. It also helps to strengthen and relax the calf muscle. The adrenal glands, which are related to the calf muscle, are also affected.
Positioning: Sit, Japanese style, at the receiver's feet.
Procedure: Squeeze the entire length of the Achilles tendon by using the index finger and the thumb. As you continue up the calf, to just above the knee joint, squeeze the large muscles of the lower leg.
Repetition: Squeeze the entire length of the Achilles tendon and the calf to just above the knee joint twice.
Time: Hold each squeeze for 3 seconds. The entire technique done twice, will take 30 seconds.

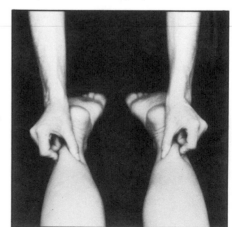

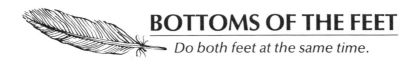

BOTTOMS OF THE FEET

Do both feet at the same time.

15) BOTTOM OF THE FOOT ACKNOWLEDGMENT

Purpose: This technique loosens the feet and prepares them for specific pressure point therapy.
Positioning: Sit, Japanese style, at receiver's feet.
Procedure: Use your thumbs to firmly massage the entire bottoms of the receiver's feet. Let your thumbs move freely. Keep them flexible and

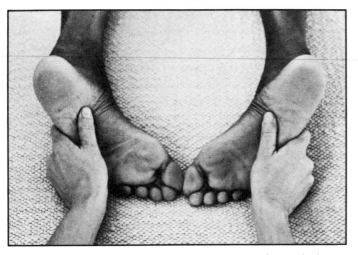

in constant motion. Do not get specific with this technique. It is a general massage technique designed primarily to relax the feet before specific pressure point therapy.
Repetition: Two or three times.
Time: 30 seconds.

16) HEEL TWIST

Purpose: This technique helps to stimulate the flow of fresh blood into the feet and to release tension from the feet and ankles.

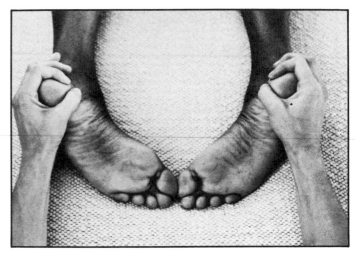

Positioning: Sit at the receiver's feet.
Procedure: Grasp both heels, hold them firmly, and simultaneously twist them first inward and then outward.
Repetition: Repeat three times in each direction.
Time: 10 seconds.

It is important to be familiar with the skeletal structure of the feet when applying heavy pressure.

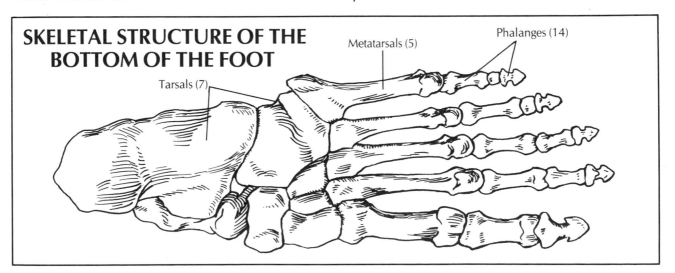

SKELETAL STRUCTURE OF THE BOTTOM OF THE FOOT

Metatarsals (5)

Phalanges (14)

Tarsals (7)

17) SQUEEZE & TWIST EDGE OF FOOT

Purpose: This regenerates the nervous system.
Positioning: Sit, at the receiver's feet.
Procedure: Begin this technique near the heel of the outside edge of the foot, and then continue

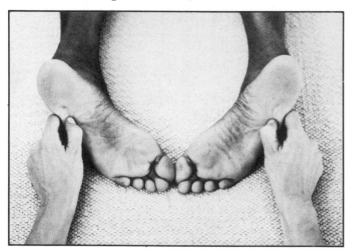

down the edge of the foot to the toes. Take some flesh between your thumb and index finger. Squeeze and gently twist the skin.
Repetition: None.
Time: 10 seconds.

18) OUTER EDGE OF THE FOOT PRESSURE

Purpose: This technique regenerates the nervous system. It is also helpful with shoulder, arm, elbow, hip and knee conditions. Hemorrhoids, too, respond to pressure applied to the back of the heel. Many people feel tingles up and down the spine during this technique. This feeling is the movement of nerve energy along the spinal column.

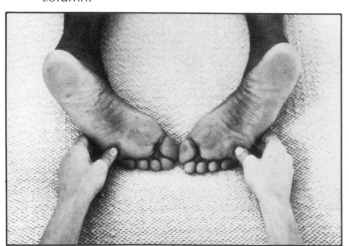

Positioning: Sit, at the receiver's feet.
Procedure: Apply a firm penetrating thumb pressure to both feet at the same time. Begin under the small toe and work your way up and around to the heel.
Repetition: Unnecessary.
Time: Hold each pressure point for 3-5 seconds. The entire technique will take 35 seconds.

19) BOTTOMS OF THE FEET PRESSURE POINTS

Purpose: Pressure applied to the related organ points on the soles of the feet stimulates the nerve endings, which, in turn, stimulate the entire nerve and its associated organs and muscles. This stimulation encourages the body's natural healing mechanism to take control and begins to right most conditions of ill health. The toxins that accumulate in the feet are released, and the general health and condition of the nerves are improved. So is the overall health of the receiver.
Positioning: Sit, at the receiver's feet.
Procedure: Apply firm pressure with your thumbs or knuckles to each of the diagnostic points. Hold pressure for 3-5 seconds. When applying pressure, direct your thoughts to the organ related to the reflex point. Try to visualize the organ. Concentration will accomplish greater results than will an absent-minded pressure.
Repetition: If any of the reflex points feels painful or tender, repeat the pressure on that point. The repetition must be gentler than the first application. The purpose is to soothe the area and give the tender reflex point the one more application of pressure needed to complete the triggering of the body's natural healing mechanism.
Time: 60 seconds.

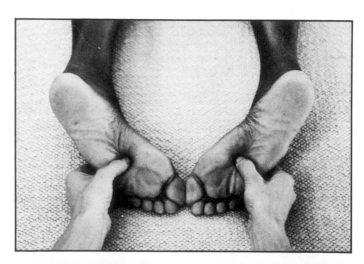

FOOT REFLEXOLOGY

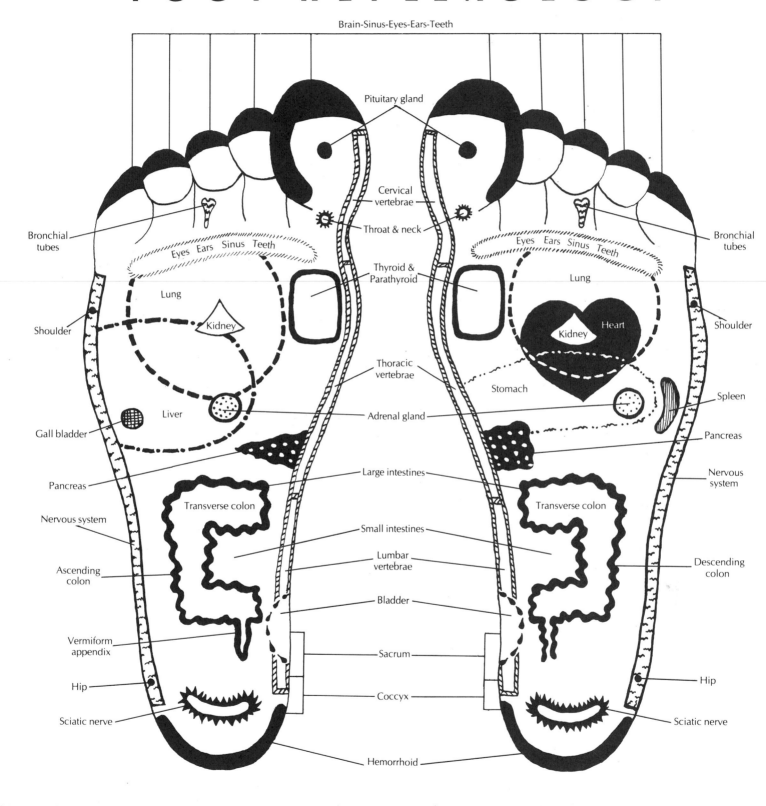

Brain-Sinus-Eyes-Ears-Teeth

Pituitary gland

Cervical vertebrae

Throat & neck

Thyroid & Parathyroid

Bronchial tubes

Eyes Ears Sinus Teeth

Lung

Shoulder

Kidney

Heart

Kidney

Lung

Eyes Ears Sinus Teeth

Bronchial tubes

Shoulder

Thoracic vertebrae

Stomach

Spleen

Gall bladder

Liver

Adrenal gland

Pancreas

Pancreas

Large intestines

Nervous system

Nervous system

Transverse colon

Transverse colon

Ascending colon

Small intestines

Lumbar vertebrae

Descending colon

Vermiform appendix

Bladder

Hip

Sacrum

Hip

Sciatic nerve

Coccyx

Sciatic nerve

Hemorrhoid

RIGHT

LEFT

67

20) TOE PAD PRESSURE, MASSAGE & SQUEEZE

Purpose: Massaging and squeezing the toes improves sinus conditions and relieves brain fatigue. Slow learners or mentally overworked individuals will benefit from this technique.

Positioning: Sit, at the receiver's feet.

Procedure: Use your thumbs to apply a firm pressure to the pads of the toes. Begin with the little toe on each foot, then work your way toward the big toe. Squeeze the sides, top and bottom of each toe.

Repetition: Repeat these techniques if the receiver is frequently troubled with sinus conditions or brain fatigue.

Time: 45 seconds.

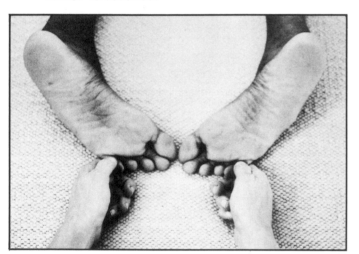

21) HEEL PRESSURE FOR SCIATIC NERVE

Purpose: This technique relieves sciatic nerve pain.

Positioning: Sit at the receiver's feet.

Procedure: Apply heavy thumb or knuckle pressure to the middle of the heel area.

Repetition: Repeat as often as necessary to relieve acute pain. If there is no pain but you wish to help cure a chronic sciatic condition, apply pressure four times to each heel.

Time: Hold each pressure point 3-5 seconds, for a total of approximately 15 seconds.

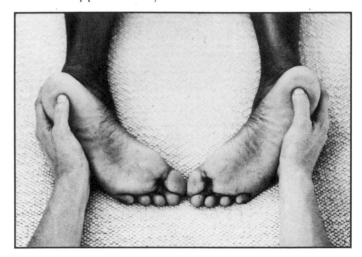

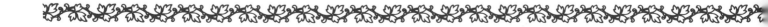

SHOULDER AND UPPER BACK

22) SHOULDER SHRUG

Purpose: Use in alternation with Technique #23 to encourage the relaxation of the shoulder and upper arm muscles.
Positioning: Sit at receiver's head.
Procedure: Massage the deltoid muscle, then grasp the top of the arms and pull the shoulders

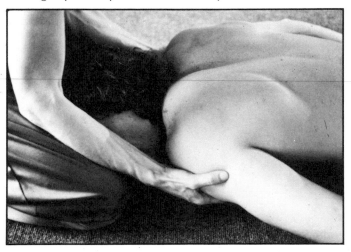

up toward the head. Use Shoulder Slide Technique #23 to return the shoulders to their normal position.
Repetition: Repeat the Shoulder Shrug two times, but alternate each shrug with Technique #23.
Time: See Technique #23.

23) SHOULDER SLIDE

Purpose: Most people hold their shoulders somewhere in the vicinity of their ears. This may be a slight exaggeration, but the fact is that many people do have a great deal of tension stored in their shoulders. Eventually, chronic neck and shoulder tension will permanently alter one's posture. The Shoulder Slide returns the shoulders to their correct position. This technique also enables the receiver to become aware of how high the shoulders are normally held.

Positioning: Sit at the receiver's head. Crouch so that the pressure does not strain your shoulders, but keep your spine properly aligned.
Procedure: Cradle the receiver's shoulders in the palms of your hands. Slowly slide the shoulders

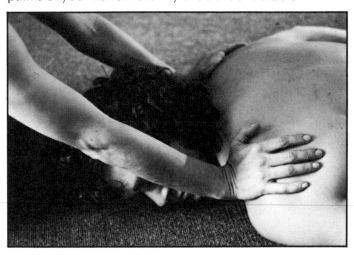

down toward the feet. Hold the shoulders in the full stretch position for 5 seconds.
Repetition: Repeat two times in alternation with Technique #22.
Time: 15 seconds.

24) SHOULDER ROTATIONS

Purpose: Shoulder Rotations relax the upper trapezius muscle and the muscles of the shoulder. They thereby release tension from the neck and the shoulders.
Positioning: There are two possible positions to assume.
1) Sit, Japanese style, at the receiver's head.
2) Kneel parallel to the receiver's body in the vicinity of the waist.
Procedure: If you assume *Position 1*, grasp both shoulders and rotate them toward you. Lift the receiver's shoulders off the mat during the motion. If the receiver is of normal weight and delicate-boned, you will be able to rotate both shoulders simultaneously.

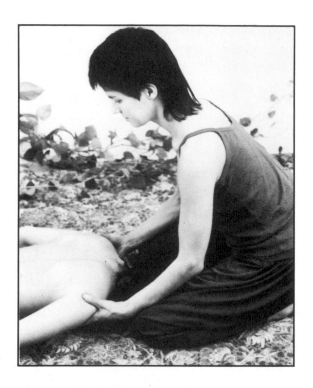

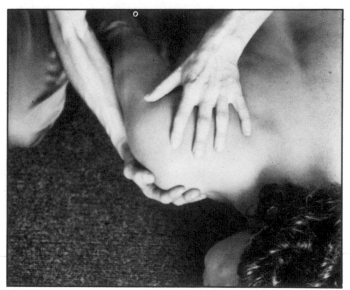

If you assume *Position 2,* slide one arm under the receiver's arm and shoulder. Use your other hand to cup the same shoulder. Now, use your arms and hands to rotate the shoulder. Rotate clockwise and counter-clockwise three times in each direction. Repeat procedure on receiver's other shoulder.
Repetition: If the receiver has chronic shoulder tension or pain, increase the number of rotations.
Time: Allow 5 seconds.

25) UPPER THORACIC VERTEBRAE TECHNIQUE

Purpose: This technique relaxes the muscles of the upper back and shoulders. The lungs, thyroid, eyes, ears, heart and stomach benefit greatly from the applications of this procedure. Also, pressure is relieved on the nerves as they emerge from the spinal column.
Positioning: Sit, Japanese style, at the receiver's head.
Procedure: Begin on either side of and between the fourth and fifth thoracic vetebrae. Execute in the same three phases as Technique #6, Vertebrae Technique.

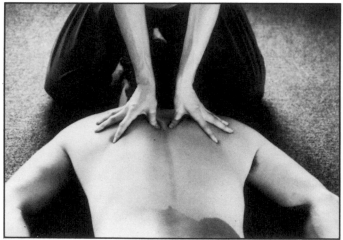

Repetition:
Phase 1: Massage between and on either side of the vertebrae three to five times by applying medium pressure with your thumbs.
Phase 2: Apply thumb pressure for 3-5 seconds to the same areas. If an area is particularly painful, repeat pressure.
Phase 3: Massage the same areas three to five times with your thumbs applying light pressure. "Make Nice."
See the photographs for Technique #6 on page 59
Time: 60 seconds.

26) UPPER TRAPEZIUS SHOULDER PRESS

Purpose: The upper trapezius, the most prominent muscle of the shoulder, is often weak or tense. This technique is designed to release tension from this muscle.

Positioning: Sit, Japanese style, at the receiver's head. Lower your torso in order to facilitate the correct application of the pressure.

Procedure: Begin at the outer edge of the shoulders, between the clavicle and the spine of the scapula. Use thumb pressure along the fullest part

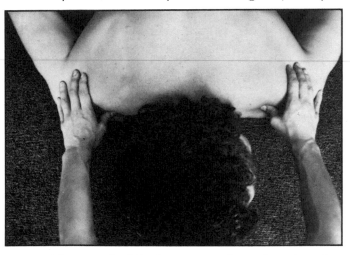

of the muscle. Work your way from the edge of the shoulders toward the vertebrae of the neck. Return to the outer edge of the shoulders. Repeat the thumb pressure along the same area. The pressure must be firm and sensitive. Most people will experience pain with these points. Do not jab your thumbs into the muscle tissue. Penetrate slowly and firmly.

Repetition: If the receiver experiences chronic shoulder tension, repeat this technique after Technique #27.

Time: Hold each thumb application of pressure for 3-5 seconds. The entire technique will take 25 seconds.

27) UPPER TRAPEZIUS SHOULDER SQUEEZE & MASSAGE

Purpose: The Shoulder Squeeze improves the flow of blood to the muscles being massaged and releases pockets of tension. It feels very good.

Positioning: Sit, Japanese style, at the receiver's head.

Procedure: Using your fingers and thumbs, massage with great compassion because a great deal of tension is stored in the shoulders. If a puffy, lumpy area comes to your attention, you have

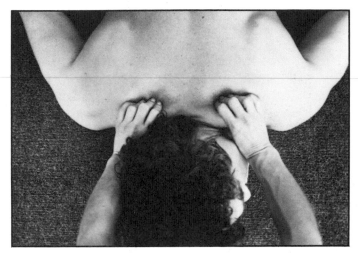

found an energy blockage or tension pocket. Concentrate on these areas, and alternate a gentle massaging motion with a delicate squeezing one. Energy blockages or tension pockets can also be dispersed by applying a gentle, but firm thumb pressure directly to the site of the blockage.

Repetition: Thumb pressure applied directly to the site of a blockage must be held for 5-7 seconds. Repeat massaging and squeezing many times.

Time: The entire technique, including massaging, thumb pressure and squeezing, will require 30 seconds.

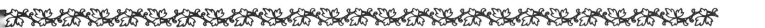

28) SHOULDER KNEADING

Purpose: Kneading releases tension and helps to free blockages in the shoulders.
Positioning: Sit, Japanese style, at receiver's head.
Procedure: Use the heels of both of your hands. Knead the part of the shoulders that is farthest

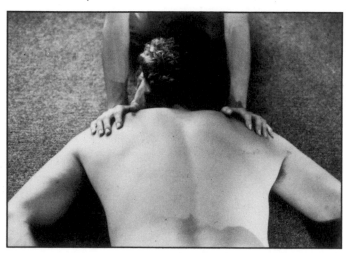

from the neck by alternating your pressure from the right to left heel. Knead *slowly* so that the rhythm established feels like a rocking, soothing motion.
Repetition: Knead each shoulder a total of five times.
Time: 10 seconds.

29) SPINAL SWEEP

Purpose: This technique provides a nice farewell to the spine before moving on to the feet. The Spinal Sweep is very relaxing.

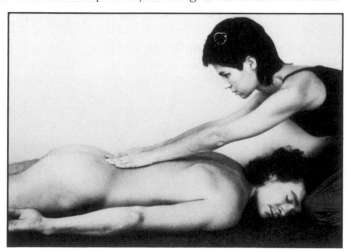

Positioning: Sit, Japanese style, at the receiver's head.
Procedure: Lay both hands flat on the sacrum. Using a medium pressure, pull your hands up along either side of the spine. As your hands reach the neck, use a lighter motion to continue the stroke up and over the neck and head.
Répetition: Repeat three times.
Time: 20 seconds.

30) FEATHERING THE SPINE

Purpose: The light gliding motion of feathering often produces goose pimples in the receiver. Feathering tells the brain to relax the area that is being feathered. Feathering is also a very quiet and gentle way to leave one part of the body for another so that the massage can continue without abrupt loss of contact.
Positioning: Sit, Japanese style, at receiver's head.
Procedure: Feather directly over the spine. Begin feathering with the right hand, then alternate with the left. Feather three inches along the coccyx with the right hand. Begin the next stroke with the left hand, but overlap by approximately one inch the area you have just feathered with the right. As you proceed, always overlap the previous area so that no part of the spine is neglected. Be sure to continue the feathering over the neck and head. Visualize that you are pulling energy up the Governing Meridian, which affects the entire spine and nervous system.
Repetition: Repeat the entire feathering of the spine two times. Complete the technique with your hands lightly resting on the receiver's head.
Time: 20 seconds.

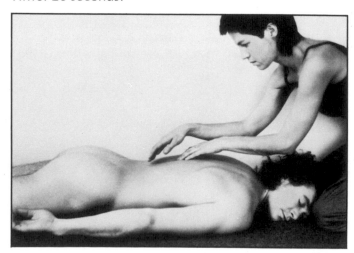

LYING SUPINE

When Technique #30 has been completed, allow 15-20 seconds for the receiver to lie comfortably relaxed. Remain seated, Japanese style, continue to hold the receiver's head loosely with both hands. Then, over a period of 30 seconds, slowly, gradually and imperceptibly draw your hands away from the head. The withdrawal must be slow so that you do not startle the receiver. This gradual departure from the body leaves the receiver feeling calm, safe and often asleep. Use a light touch and a soft voice to bring the receiver back from a sleep state. Suggest that the receiver turn over when ready and able. Even if the receiver is not asleep, use this method to leave the body and reestablish verbal communication.

A few adjustments must be made to assure the receiver's comfort while lying supine.
A) Place one folded bed pillow under each leg. The pillow raises the legs slightly and thus takes pressure off the lower back. People who suffer from chronic low back pain will appreciate the relief. Those who do not will receive a more relaxed massage.

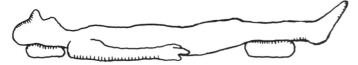

B) Squat at the receiver's head. Place both hands and arms under the shoulders and partially under the back. Take hold of the back and stretch it toward you. Stretching the spine eliminates the exaggerated arch of the lower back, which is the result of weak abdominals and tense lower back muscles. Stretching and flattening the back allows it to assume a more correct alignment. Receiving

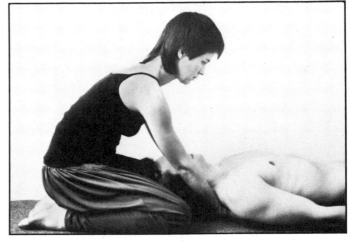

a massage in a stretched, relaxed position with the spine properly aligned enables the body to release more tension.

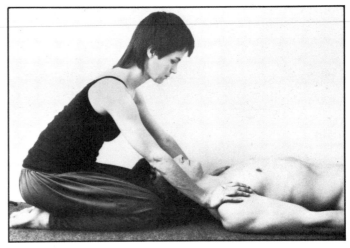

C) Cup the shoulders and push them down toward the receiver's toes.
D) Grasp the underside of the receiver's head and neck, then stretch and pull the head and neck toward you. Repeat this stretching and pulling three times.

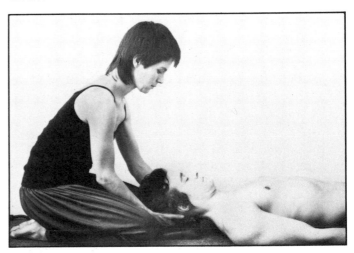

73

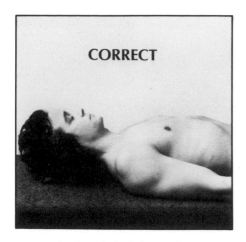

CORRECT

E) Next, raise the head slightly and insert a thin pillow under the occipital protuberance, which is the big bump at the back of the head. If you do not have a tiny pillow, use a towel that has been folded tightly. The aim is to raise the head about 1½-2 inches off the mat. The following photograph shows that when the head lies on the mat, it tends to tilt up and back. This tilt puts pressure on

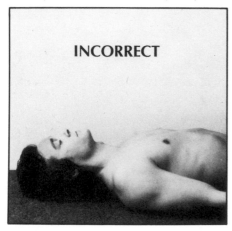

INCORRECT

the first few cervical vertebrae and increases tension in the shoulders and neck. Once the head is on the pillow, insert your fingers under the base of the skull and again stretch the neck toward you. Rest the receiver's head, with the neck in the stretched position, on the pillow. Be sure the chin is not sticking up in the air. In this position much of the tension in the neck and shoulders will automatically be released as you massage the rest of the body. Indeed, by the time you begin massaging the neck, much of the blockage and pain has already been relieved.

F) Cover the receiver if the possibility of a chill exists. Use a sheet in warm weather and an electric blanket when the air is cool or cold.

G) If the receiver feels any tension or pain in the neck or shoulders as a result of lying in the prone position for the back work, massage the neck and shoulders for one or two minutes by using Techniques #69 and #71. These techniques will release any discomfort and allow you to proceed to THE FEET PART II.

Time: 4 minutes.

TOP OF THE FEET

31) GENERAL FOOT ACKNOWLEDGMENT (BOTH FEET)

Purpose: This technique loosens and relaxes the feet before the application of specific pressure point techniques. A brief, gentle massage before beginning to apply heavy pressure enables the feet to enjoy the firmer pressure.

Positioning: Sit, at the receiver's feet.

Procedure: Acknowledge the entire foot by massaging it with gentle pressure and by lightly stroking and bending the foot.

Repetition: Unnecessary

Time: 30 seconds.

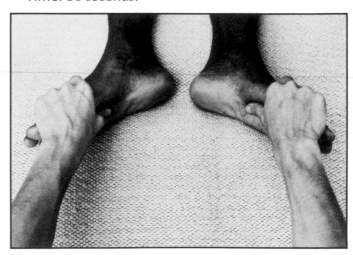

32) PULL AND MASSAGE TOES (BOTH FEET)

Purpose: Massaging and pulling the toes helps to loosen each toe. This technique also returns stagnant blood to the heart and thus allows fresh blood to flow to the toes. When you consider the shoes we wear, especially those worn by women, it is easy to understand why massaging and pulling the toes feels so good and relieves so much pain. Manipulation of the toes also indirectly moves the metatarsal bones and helps to loosen the bones and muscles of the foot itself. Furthermore, toe manipulation helps to improve sinus conditions and brain fatigue as well as other brain-related conditions.

Positioning: Remain seated, Japanese style, at the feet.

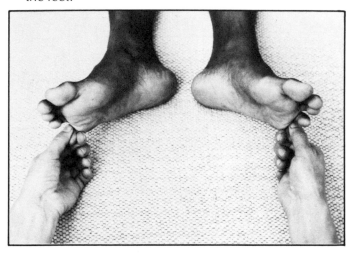

Procedure: Begin massaging the small toes. Methodically, toe by toe, work your way to the big toes. Manipulate the same toes on each foot at the same time. Squeeze and massage each toe from the tip of its nail to the base where it joins the foot. Massaging from the base of the toe to the tip of the nail does not return as much stagnant blood to the heart for recirculation. After you have massaged one pair of toes, give the same toes a firm, but gentle pull and twist to stretch and further relax them.

Repetition: Unnecessary.

Time: Allow 10 seconds for each pair of toes. The total time will be approximately 50 seconds.

33) ANKLE ROTATIONS (ONE FOOT)

Purpose: These rotations relax the joint and increase the flexibility of the ankle. In addition to improving blood and lymph circulation, this technique frees stagnant meridian energy trapped in the ankles.

Positioning: Sit, Japanese style, at the receiver's side. Position yourself perpendicular to the calf muscles.

Procedure: Grasp the ball of the foot. Rest the receiver's lower leg over your knees. Be sure the ankle and foot do not make contact with your legs. With the palm of one hand, hold the bottom of the receiver's foot. With your other hand, support the leg just above the ankle. Make three large, slow rotations, first to the right and then to the left.

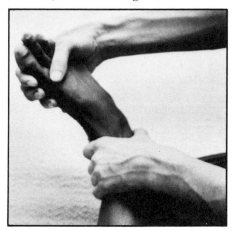

Repetition: Complete all three rotations in one direction before rotating in the other direction.

Time: 10 seconds per foot.

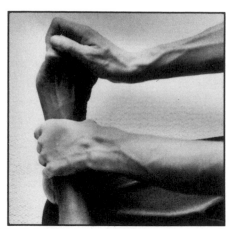

34) FIVE-TOE ROTATION (ONE FOOT)

Purpose: This technique further loosens cramped toes and metatarsal bones.

Positioning: Same as technique #33.

Procedure: Grasp the foot with one hand and hold the toes with the other hand. Slowly rotate all five toes at once.

Repetition: Rotate three times to the right and then to the left.

Time: 5 seconds per foot.

35) INDIVIDUAL TOE ROTATIONS AND PULLS (ONE FOOT)

Purpose: This technique continues to loosen cramped and tense toes. It also improves sinus conditions and brain fatigue.

Positioning: Same as technique #33.

Procedure: Rotate each toe. Rotate it in both directions, and then pull the toe firmly while twisting it slightly. You may hear a popping sound coming from the toes. This is a good sound, for it indicates that the toe joint has been released. Most people enjoy toe rotations and pulls, although some find it very unpleasant and even

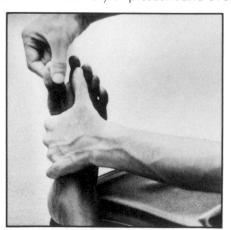

painful. If you sense discomfort on the part of the receiver, *gently* rotate and *lightly* stretch the toes. Do not force them to tolerate a more firmly executed pull and twist. Remember that pain is not the object and that excellent results can be achieved without causing excess discomfort.

Repetition: Rotate each toe twice in both directions, then twist as you pull. If you do not get the desired popping sound, try to pull the toe once more. If, however, it does not come easily the second time, move on to the next toe.

Time: Allow approximately 10 seconds per toe and a total of 50 seconds per foot.

36) ARCH PRESSURE FOR THE SPINE (ONE FOOT)

Purpose: Pressure along the arch of the foot helps to relieve back pain. Tension and spasms both respond quite quickly to these reflex points. If the receiver experiences occasional back pain, but is not feeling pain at the time of the massage, this technique will help discourage the return of the pain. Also it will ultimately help to correct the condition. Acute back pain, the sort that occurs suddenly because of a fall or because of lifting a heavy object, responds very well to these pressure points. Pressure along the arch of the foot also helps to rejuvenate the entire nervous system.

Positioning: Sit, Japanese style, at the receiver's head.

Procedure: Apply firm pressure from the outside base of the big toe nail, then along the arch of the foot to the back of the heel. Use the tip of your

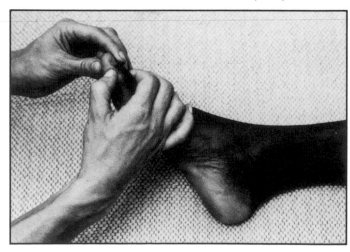

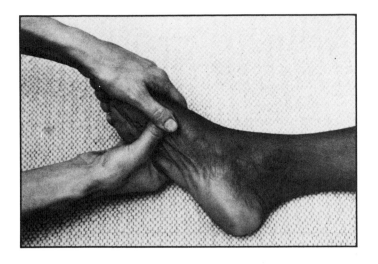

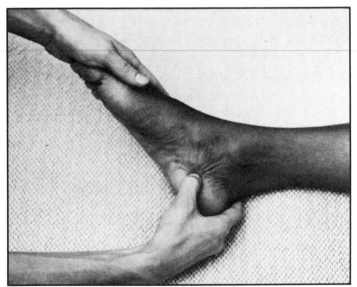

37) KIDNEY & SEXUAL/ REPRODUCTIVE ORGANS MASSAGE (ONE FOOT)

Purpose: Points corresponding to the kidneys and sexual organs are located in approximately the same place. Pressure applied to the appropriate area will assist the kidneys in their eliminative processes and will tone up the sexual organs of both males and females. Reproductive, menstrual, prostate and other sexual organ malfunctioning can be corrected by regular applications of pressure to these reflex points.

Positioning: Sit, Japanese style, at the receiver's feet.

Procedure: Holding one of the receiver's feet in your hand, apply several applications of firm pressure to the hollow area just below the inside of the anklebone.

Repetition: Repeat only if the receiver has any condition that these points will help.

Time: Approximately 10 seconds per foot.

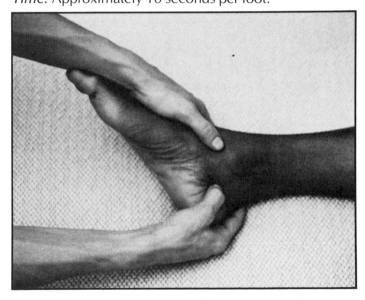

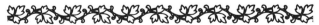

thumb to apply firm pressure from the base of the nail until you pass the sesamoid bone, which is the large bony protrusion on the bottom of the foot under the big toe. Next, using the ball of one thumb and assisting with your other thumb, apply firm, lingering pressure from the sesamoid bone to the heel. Use the tip-of-the-thumb technique for the heel. Don't skip any area of the arch. Apply pressure to every inch of the entire area discussed.

Repetition: If the receiver has back pain when you begin the massage, several applications will be necessary to relieve it. Otherwise, once down the toe, arch and heel is sufficient.

Time: Hold each pressure application for 3-5 seconds. Total time amounts to 50 seconds per foot.

38) ANKLEBONE MASSAGE (ONE FOOT)

Purpose: Massaging directly around the anklebone will benefit the male and female reproductive organs. It also feels really nice.

Positioning: Sit, Japanese style, at the receiver's feet.

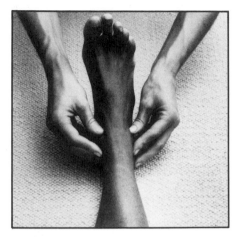

Procedure: Cup the fingers and thumb of each hand around the anklebones of one foot. Massage the area by moving all the fingers and your thumbs in unison. Stay close to the anklebone.

Repetition: Repeat only if the receiver's condition warrants continued use of these points.

Time: 5 seconds per foot.

39) ANKLE LYMPHATIC MASSAGE (BOTH FEET)

Purpose: This procedure flushes the lymphatic system at the ankle and moves along the stagnant toxins. Lymph tends to stagnate in the feet because most of us lead sedentary lives and have poor circulation

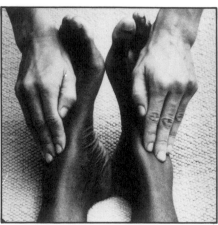

Positioning: Sit, Japanese style, at the receiver's feet.

Procedure: Use four fingers in a back-and-forth motion. Put most of your force in the forward motion so that the toxins will flush away from the feet. Gently bring your fingers back in preparation for the next motion forward. Do both feet at the same time.

Repetition: Use five firm motions backed up with five light gliding motions.

Time: 5 seconds.

40) FOUR FINGER METATARSAL SLIDE (BOTH FEET)

Purpose: Sliding your fingers along the grooves of the metatarsal bones is a very pleasurable sensation. This technique sends energy to the chest, lung and breast area. Any condition relating to this area of the body will heal itself more quickly with repeated use of these points.

Positioning: Sit, Japanese style, at the receiver's feet.

Procedure: Position the four fingers of both hands in the grooves of the metatarsal bones at the base of the toes on the top of both feet. Firmly force your fingers into these grooves while slowly and firmly sliding them toward and over the ankle. The technique is more pleasurable if the motion continues up and over the ankle. As the metatarsal bones do not extend to the ankle, you will loosen the grooves, but the pleasurable skin sensations derived from the pressure of the fingers sliding up and over the ankle warrants its continuation.

Repetition: Repeat three times on both feet at the same time.

Time: A total of 10 seconds is required.

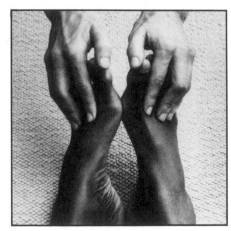

41) TOP OF THE FOOT TWIST (ONE FOOT)

Purpose: This twist relaxes the foot.
Positioning: Sit between the receiver's feet.
Procedure: Grasping the foot with both hands, twist your hands in opposite directions up and down the foot.

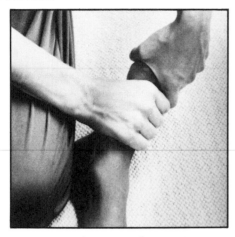

Repetition: Twist the entire foot twice.
Time: 7 seconds per foot.

At this point you have completed a thorough massage of one foot. Repeat Techniques #33 through #38, and #41, on the other foot. Then proceed to Technique #42.

FOOT REFLEXOLOGY SIDE VIEWS

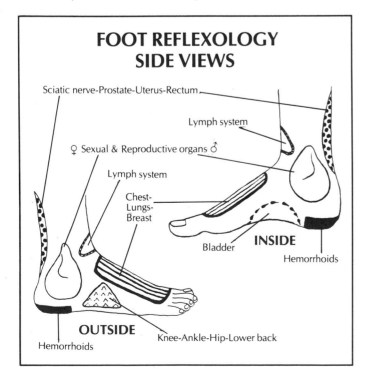

Sciatic nerve-Prostate-Uterus-Rectum

Lymph system

♀ Sexual & Reproductive organs ♂

Lymph system

Chest-Lungs-Breast

Bladder

INSIDE

Hemorrhoids

OUTSIDE

Hemorrhoids

Knee-Ankle-Hip-Lower back

FRONT OF THE LEGS

42) LIVER AID

Purpose: Applying pressure to the liver points along the shinbone will assist the liver in the performance of its 500 known functions. An extremely overworked organ, the liver can use all the help it can get. People who drink a lot of alcohol will find these points particularly useful.
Positioning: Sit, Japanese style, slightly between the receiver's legs.
Procedure: Begin at the ankle. Apply firm 3-second thumb pressure in the designated places as you move up the shinbone.

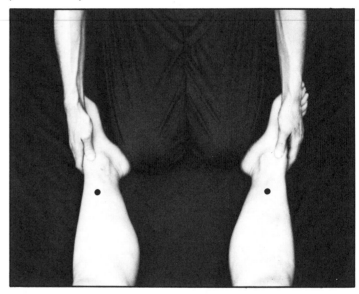

Repetition: No repetition is necessary unless a known liver condition or weakness exists. In such a case, repeat pressure to all the points three times and hold each point for ten seconds.
Time: 10 seconds, if no known condition exists.

43) KNEE LYMPHATIC MASSAGE

Purpose: This technique clears the lymph nodes that cluster around the knee and helps to strengthen the tendons of the muscles that insert around the knee. Knee pain also responds to this technique.

Positioning: Sit, Japanese style, between the receiver's open legs.

Procedure: Using four fingers and a circular massaging motion, massage around both knees at the same time. If knee problems exist, use firm thumb pressure on the same area after the four-finger massage. Do not directly massage the patella, or knee cap, as this does not feel good to the receiver. When applying firm thumb pressure, penetrate slowly so that you can clearly determine the bony structure under the skin. If pressure is ap-

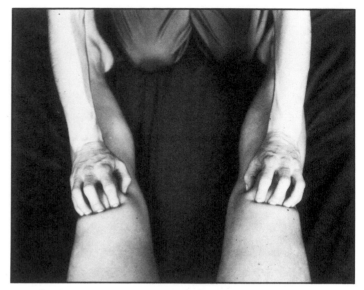

plied too quickly, you will not be fully aware of the underlying bone structure and may very well slip and hurt the receiver.

Repetition: Massage each area with four fingers five times. When applying thumb pressure, hold each pressure application for 3-5 seconds.

Time: 30 seconds.

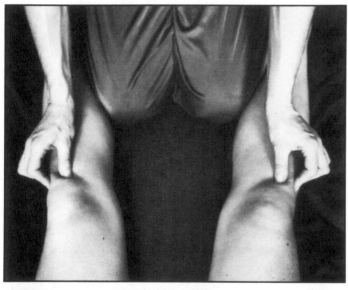

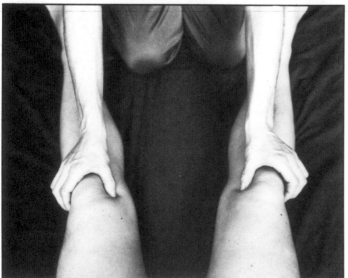

44) THIGH LYMPHATIC FLUSH

Purpose: The Thigh Lymphatic Flush is useful for several conditions. Primarily it improves the functioning of the small and large intestines as well as that of the sexual and reproductive organs. Massaging the inside of the thigh also affects the tone and functioning of the abdominal muscles, the hamstrings and the quadratus lumborum. Low back pain, headaches and hemorrhoids also respond to thigh massage and manipulation. Massaging the outside of the thigh helps to alleviate breast and chest pain before, during and after menstruation. It is also very stimulating and beneficial to the colon. Constipation, diarrhea and other colon conditions respond favorably to the massaging of these points on a regular basis.

Positioning: Kneel below the receiver's knee with your knees on either side of the receiver's leg. Do not sit on the leg, for it may be uncomfortable for the receiver to bear the pressure of your body weight.

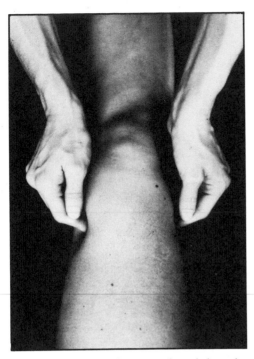

Procedure: Place four fingers of each hand on either side of one thigh beside the knee. Massage one leg at a time. Use a progressive, circular massaging motion as you work your way up the thigh. Use medium to firm pressure. Proceed with great compassion, for this area is very often tender.

Repetition: Repeat two times, more often if a problem relating to these lymphatic massage areas exists.

Time: 60 seconds.

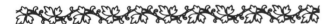

45) THIGH TWIST

Purpose: The Thigh Twist feels terrific. This technique stimulates circulation to the thigh and gives its meridians a twist that helps to improve their energy flow. The meridians involved are those of the liver, kidney, spleen, gall bladder and stomach.

Positioning: Spread the receiver's legs open and straddle the leg opposite to the one you are twisting.

Procedure: Start near the knee and twist your way up the thigh. Place one hand on the inside of the thigh and the other on the outside. As you push away from you and into the thigh with one hand, pull toward you with the other hand. Incorporate a slight twist to the push-and-pull motion. After one area of the thigh has been twisted, move slightly farther up the thigh and repeat the technique, but this time switch hands. Place the hand that was on the inside of the thigh on the outside of the thigh and the hand that was on the outside of the thigh on the inside of the thigh. Also, push with the hand that was pulling and pull with the hand that was pushing. By switching hands and by alternating the push and pull, you can provide the thigh with a better twist. Use the heel of your hand along with the full hand to apply the push so as to achieve more strength and a better twist with less effort. Work slowly.

Repetition: Repeat twice because it feels oh so good!

Time: 30 seconds for both legs.

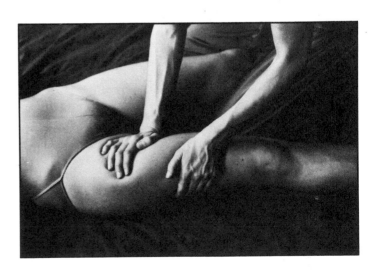

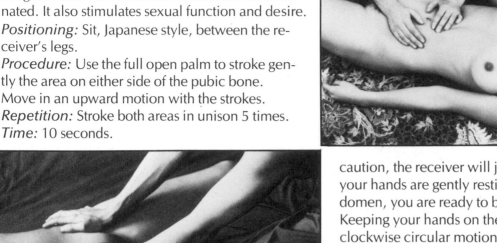

46) PUBIC LYMPH DRAINAGE

Purpose: This technique forces the lymph fluid of the groin area into the chest where it can be eliminated. It also stimulates sexual function and desire.
Positioning: Sit, Japanese style, between the receiver's legs.
Procedure: Use the full open palm to stroke gently the area on either side of the pubic bone. Move in an upward motion with the strokes.
Repetition: Stroke both areas in unison 5 times.
Time: 10 seconds.

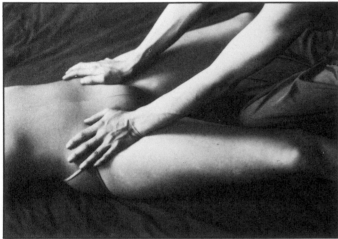

caution, the receiver will jump with a start. Once your hands are gently resting on the receiver's abdomen, you are ready to begin the technique. Keeping your hands on the abdomen, begin a clockwise circular motion. Move from the lower right side of the abdomen up, across and down the left side of the abdomen. Use two hands, one after the other following the direction of movement of feces.
Repetition: Repeat three to five times.
Time: 10 seconds.

THE TORSO

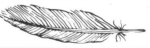

47) ABDOMINAL/COLON MASSAGE

Purpose: This technique helps to relieve constipation and brings fresh blood to the abdominal area. The internal organs thus receive fresh blood and nutrients to help improve their functioning.
Positioning: Sit, Japanese style, at the receiver's waist. The side of your leg should be touching the receiver's body. Do not lean into the receiver as you work, as your body weight will become very heavy and uncomfortable.
Procedure: Sit at the receiver's side. *Gently* lay both hands on the abdomen with extreme tenderness, for this part of the body is especially vulnerable. Unless you proceed with the utmost

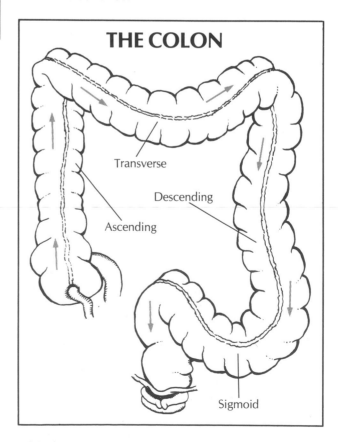

THE COLON

Transverse

Descending

Ascending

Sigmoid

48) BOWEL STIMULATION

Purpose: This technique stimulates the peristaltic motion of the large intestine.

Positioning: Sit, Japanese style, at the receiver's side.

Procedure: Begin at the lower right side of the abdomen. Lay your right hand gently over the abdomen and gradually increase its application of pressure. A light to medium pressure is all that is necessary. Next position the four fingers of your left hand between your right thumb and index finger. Gently and slowly insert your fingers into the abdomen. Watch the receiver's face for any grimace that will indicate you are penetrating too deeply. The secret is to penetrate *very* slowly and *very* gently. If the receiver's body senses that you are moving carefully, it will relax and open up to you, and you will not cause discomfort. Repeat the same technique up the right side of the colon, then across the transverse colon and down the descending colon on the left side of the abdomen. When you reach the lower left side, hold the last penetration a little longer than the others. Complete the last penetration by vibrating your hand and arm so that the vibrations extend through your fingers into the receiver's abdomen.

Repetition: No repetition is necessary. If the receiver suffers from chronic constipation, repeat the final penetration and vibration three times. Always apply penetrating force in the direction of the movement of the feces in the bowels.

Time: Hold the penetrations for the ascending, transverse and descending colons for 3 seconds. Hold the final penetration for 5 seconds and vibrate for 5 seconds. Total time: 40 seconds.

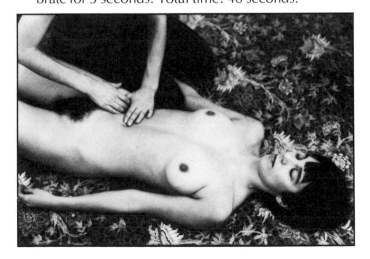

49) WAIST LIFT

Purpose: This technique trims the waistline and stimulates functions of the liver and gall bladder.

Positioning: Straddle the receiver. Your feet should be near the waist and hips. Bend over, but be sure to keep your back correctly aligned. Insert your hands under the arch of the receiver's back.

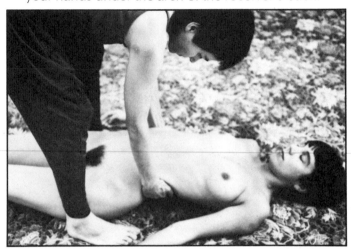

Procedure: Bending over the receiver with your feet on either side of the body and your hands inserted under the arch of the body, lift and pull. Bend your knees as you execute this technique to relieve the strain on your lower back. If you are strong enough, lift the receiver's body partially off the mat. Don't be concerned if you are not. It is sufficient simply to lift the flesh of the waist up off the mat. This technique feels better if executed slowly.

Repetition: Repeat three times.

Time: 15 seconds.

50) LYMPHATIC FINGER FLUSH

Purpose: This technique releases stagnant lymphatic fluids from the lymph nodes located between the ribs. It also aids digestion and stimulates the internal muscles between the ribs.

Positioning: Straddle the receiver with your feet on either side of their waist, or else kneel at receiver's waist.

Procedure: Begin on the side of the rib cage near the waist. Insert your fingers into the intercostal spaces between the ribs. Apply enough pressure

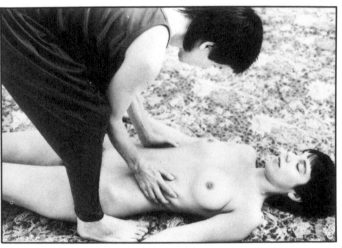

to fit your fingers snugly between the ribs, and continue to apply pressure as you pull the fingers up the side of the body onto the chest. Try to keep the fingers in the intercostal spaces between the ribs, but don't worry if one finger slips out here and there. It's the overall effect that counts. Continue this technique all the way up the chest to the breast.

Repetition: Repeat the technique twice for each area of the ribs.

Time: 15 seconds.

51) LIVER & STOMACH LYMPHATIC DRAINAGE

Purpose: This technique improves the functioning of the liver and the stomach. It thus provides an invaluable aid to digestion.

Positioning: Sit, Japanese style, at the receiver's side.

Procedure: Insert your thumbs in the intercostal space between the fifth and sixth ribs on both

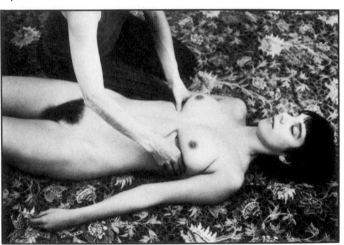

sides of the sternum. Begin near the sternum. Using tiny circular motions, massage the space between the ribs. Locate this intercostal space, which is directly under the breast line in women and directly under the pectoralis major sternal muscle in men, and then massage both sides at the same time. Massage from the sternum to beyond the nipple on the side of the chest.

Repetition: Massage each area of the intercostal space between the fifth and sixth ribs with three circular motions, then move on to the next area between the same ribs.

Time: 15 seconds.

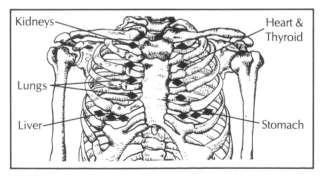

52) LUNG LYMPHATIC DRAINAGE

Purpose: Our lungs have to cope with excessive amounts of pollution and cigarette smoke. This technique helps to relieve the lungs of some of their burden. If you are a smoker, it is wise to massage these points for one minute several times a day.

Positioning: Sit, Japanese style, at the receiver's side.

Procedure: Insert your fingers into intercostal space between the third and fourth ribs, and then the space between the fourth and fifth, on either side of the sternum. Press into these spaces firmly with a tiny, circular massaging motion.

Repetition: Massage the intercostal spaces on both sides at the same time three to five times.

Time: 10 seconds.

52

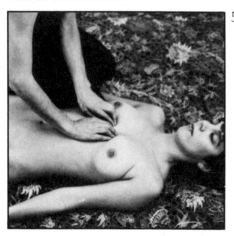

53

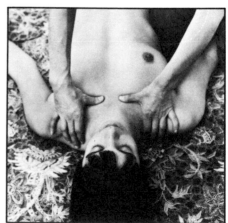

53) HEART & THYROID LYMPHATIC POINTS

Purpose: These points will help improve heart and thyroid functions. Heart problems and thyroid conditions respond to these points if they are massaged regularly.

Positioning: Sit, Japanese style, at the receiver's side.

Procedure: Insert your thumbs in the intercostal space between the second and third ribs on either side of the sternum. Use your thumbs, in a tiny, circular massaging motion. Massage near the sternum only.

Repetition: Massage the area seven times.

Time: 5 seconds.

54) KIDNEY LYMPHATIC DRAINAGE

Purpose: This technique will help improve your kidney functions. It will also help improve kidney disorders when used regularly and frequently.

Positioning: Sit, Japanese style, at the receiver's side.

Procedure: Massage directly over the first rib, which is located directly under the prominent protuberances of the clavicle bones. It is sometimes difficult to locate the first rib. Don't worry about it. Just be sure you are directly under those bony nobs at the base of the neck.

Repetition: Massage the area six or seven times with a circular motion.

Time: 10 seconds.

54

55) BREAST LUMP CHECK

Purpose: A massage is the perfect time to check the breasts for lumps. It should be done regularly, but as many women fear examining their breasts themselves, a breast check once a week during a massage is the next best thing. Early detection has saved many a breast!

Positioning: Sit, Japanese style, next to the receiver.

Procedure: A very light touch is essential. Feel the entire breast for lumps by using a gentle, small circular motion of the fingers. Also inspect the breasts for irregularity of color. Remember that just before, during and sometimes after a menstrual cycle, a woman's breasts tend to be a little lumpy because the glands are swollen. If there is a swelling, and if it does not disappear after the menstrual cycle is completed, it would be wise to visit a homoeopathic doctor. I stress homoeopathy because the herbs used by homoeopathic doctors have saved many a breast that was doomed for removal by orthodox doctors. Surgery should be considered only as a last resort. It is a well-known fact that far too many mastectomy operations are performed each year. Many breasts have been removed unnecessarily.

Repetition: Repeat only when you are uncertain.
Time: 30 seconds.

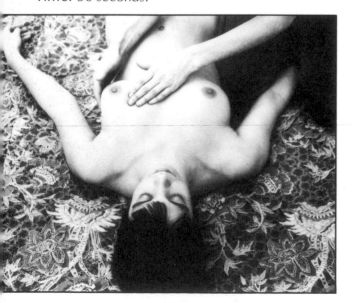

56) SHOULDER KNEADING

Purpose: Tense, raised shoulders respond very well to this technique. Slow kneading helps the shoulders to relax and loosen up. These same points also stimulate brain and lung functions.

Positioning: Kneel next to the receiver's chest and place the heel of your hands into the hollow of the receiver's shoulders.

Procedure: Slowly, but firmly, using your body weight, begin a rocking motion. Alternate your body weight between the right and left shoulders.

Repetition: Rock each shoulder five times, or rock both shoulders a total of ten times.
Time: 10 seconds.

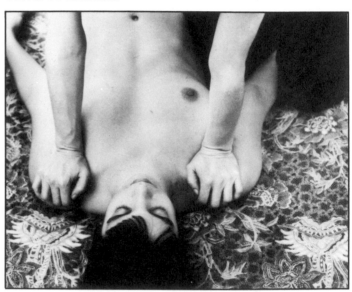

HANDS & ARMS

Do one hand and arm thoroughly before doing the other.

57) HAND FAN SPREAD

Purpose: This technique spreads open the hands to help release stored tension. It also helps to improve the flow of energy along the meridians that terminate in the hand. It thus affects the functioning of the Large Intestine, Small Intestine, Heart, Lung, Heart Constrictor, and Triple Heater/Warmer Meridians, as well as the functioning of the organs related to these meridians.

Positioning: Sit, Japanese style, at the receiver's side below the hand.

Procedure: Spread or fan the receiver's hand. Pull your thumbs first across the back of the hand, then across the palm of the hand. Do not use too much pressure, as it will feel to the receiver like you are splitting or tearing the skin of the hand.

Repetition: Repeat three times on both sides of the hand.

Time: 10 seconds.

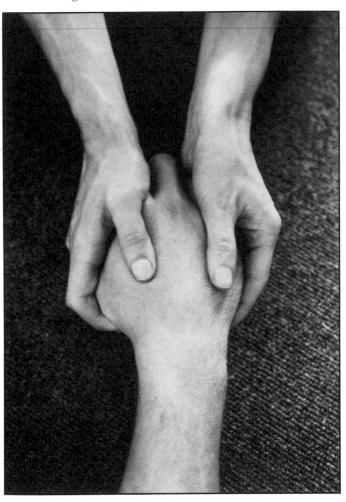

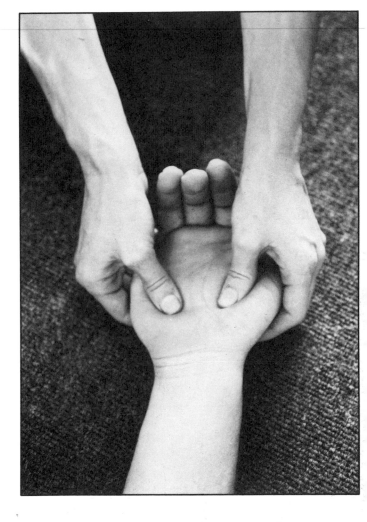

58) FINGER & THUMB MASSAGE

Purpose: This technique returns the blood of the fingers and hands to the heart. It thereby allows fresh blood to enter the fingers and hands. It also serves to stimulate the energy flow of the meridians mentioned in Technique #57.

Positioning: Sit, Japanese style, at the receiver's side.

Procedure: Begin massaging the fingers at the base of the nails. Use your thumb and index finger to apply a firm pressure to either side of the base of the nail. This technique stimulates the flow of energy in the meridian that terminates or begins in the finger you are massaging. Then, with a firm massaging and squeezing motion, move from the tip of the finger to the hand. Support the receiver's hand while massaging the fingers. Twist each finger once in both directions. If you hear a snapping or popping sound, do not be alarmed. This sound is good, for it indicates the finger joints are being released. Next, pull each finger. Repeat the same procedure for each finger and the thumb. Do not massage the other hand until you have completely finished the hand and arm on which you are working.

Repetition: No repetition is necessary.

Time: 50 seconds for each hand.

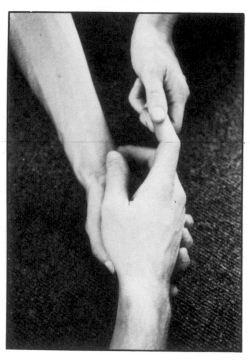

59) WRIST STRETCHES

Purpose: This technique improves the flexibility of the wrist joint, and thus the flow of energy in the meridians that travel along the arm into the hand. See Technique #57.

Positioning: Sit, Japanese style, at the receiver's side below the hand.

Procedure: Hold the receiver's arm with one of your hands. Bend the wrist backward and then forward . Next, bend the wrist to the right and then to the left. Bend gently so as not to harm the receiver.

Repetition: No repetition is necessary.

Time: 15 seconds.

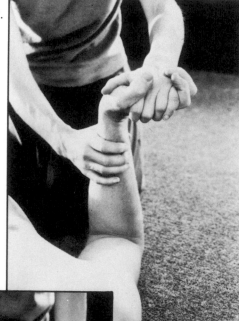

60) FOREARM MASSAGE

Purpose: This is a very general technique, its aim being to force the blood up the arm and back to the heart.

Positioning: Sit, Japanese style, next to the receiver's arm.

Procedure: Begin at the wrist. Massage up the forearm to the elbow with your thumbs on top of the forearm and your fingers on the underside. Use a squeezing and twisting forward motion as you move up from the wrist to the elbow.

Repetition: Repeat twice.

Time: 15 seconds.

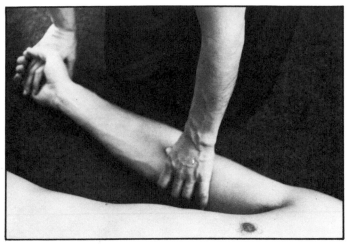

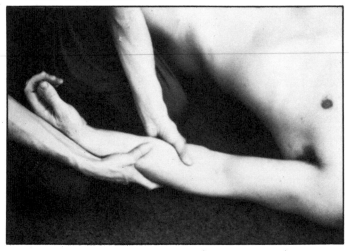

Procedure: Apply a firm, penetrating pressure to the points on all three meridians. Complete all the points of one meridian before proceeding to the next meridian. Use your thumb to apply that pressure. Be sure your posture is correct. See photograph. Your pressure must be perpendicular to the surface of the receiver's forearm so that you will not tire. Apply pressure from the crease of the elbow to the wrist.

Repetition: Hold each pressure point for 3-5 seconds. Use 5-second pressure for those meridians that you feel are most important to the receiver.

Time: 50 seconds.

61) FOREARM: LUNG—HEART CONSTRICTOR (CIRCULATION/SEX ORGANS) —HEART PRESSURE POINTS

Purpose: Pressure applied to the Lung Meridian points helps correct lung disorders. Pressure on the Heart Constrictor points directly affects the receiver's circulation and sex organs, but not the heart itself. The Heart Meridian, which lies next to the Heart Constrictor Meridian, does affect the heart organ.

Positioning: Sit, Japanese style, next to the receiver's arm.

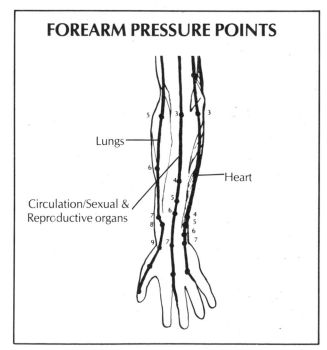

FOREARM PRESSURE POINTS

Lungs

Heart

Circulation/Sexual & Reproductive organs

62) UPPER ARM SQUEEZE & TWIST

Purpose: This technique feels absolutely wonderful, which is the main reason I employ it. Incidentally, it gives the meridians of the upper arm a good twist that enables their energy to flow more freely. It also provides the deltoids and triceps with a nice little massage that helps release some of the tension from these muscles. The meridians involved are the Heart, Lung, Heart Constrictor,

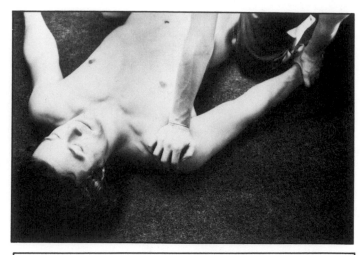

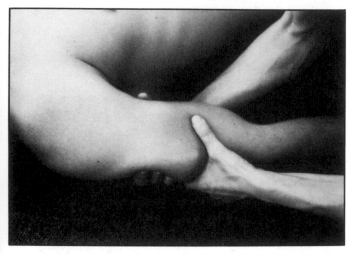

Large and Small Intestines and the Triple Warmer.
Positioning: Straddle the receiver's arm on your knees.
Procedure: Hold the receiver's arm in both your hands. Squeeze and gently knead the arm while twisting it slightly. Continue this technique up the receiver's arm to the shoulder.
Repetition: Squeeze, twist and knead each area of the arm three times.
Time: 10 seconds.

63) UPPER ARM LUNG MERIDIAN PRESSURE

Purpose: This technique improves the flow of energy along the Lung Meridian and helps correct lung disturbances.
Positioning: Execute this technique while you are still straddling the receiver's arm.
Procedure: Use the heel of your hand to apply 3-

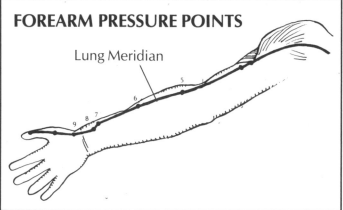

FOREARM PRESSURE POINTS

Lung Meridian

second pressure to the upper arm portion of the lung meridian. Begin on the front of the shoulder and continue down the arm to the elbow.
Repetition: No repetition is necessary.
Time: 10 seconds.

64) TRICEPS MASSAGE

Purpose: Massaging the origin and insertion of the triceps helps to strengthen the muscle, benefits the immune system and helps to regulate abnormal sugar metabolism. The triceps tends to be one of the first muscles to sag. You've all seen people with flabby arms wearing short-sleeve shirts. This muscle can be firmed and toned by regular massaging of its origin and insertion. The origins are located on the posterior shaft of the humerus and along the outside edge of the scapula. The insertion is just below the elbow on the forearm. Each muscle of the body is related to a par-

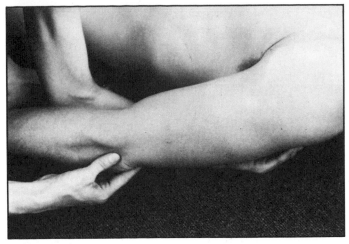

ticular organ, or organs, and is capable of affecting specific body functions. The triceps correspond to the immune system and the spleen as well as the pancreas. Most people, therefore, would benefit from regular massaging of this muscle.

Positioning: Straddle the receiver's arm. Place the fingers of one hand over the top of the humerous near the outside edge of the scapula, and place the fingers of the other hand just below the elbow bone.

Procedure: Use your fingers and a circular, firm massaging motion to thoroughly massage the origin and insertion of this muscle.

Repetition: Massage the origin and insertion of the triceps quite thoroughly.

Time: 10 seconds.

65) ARM TWIST

Purpose: The Arm Twist releases tension from the shoulder and elbow joints.

Positioning: Sit at the receiver's side below the hand.

Procedure: Holding the forearm and upper arm, gently, but firmly twist the entire arm. Twist first to the left and then to the right.

Repetition: A twist in each direction is sufficient.

Time: 5 seconds.

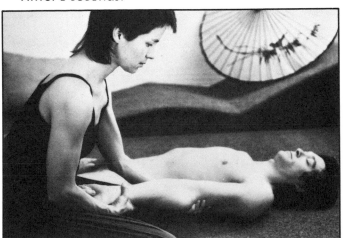

66) CROSS-OVER TECHNIQUE

Purpose: This technique makes the crossing of the body rather simple and unnoticeable. If done correctly, the receiver will not know you have proceeded to the other side of the body. Once there, you will be ready to commence work on the other arm.

Positioning: Kneel between the arm you have just massaged and the receiver's body.

Procedure: Move the receiver's opposite arm away from the body. Place the heels of your hands into the hollows of the receiver's shoulders. Gradually transfer your body weight from your knees to the heels of your hands and your feet. Using your hands as pivotal points, lift first one leg, and then the other, to the opposite side of the receiver's body. The technique is complete when you are on your knees between the receiver's opposite arm and the receiver's body.

Repetition: Unnecessary.

Time: 5 seconds.

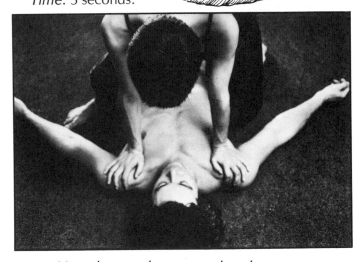

Now that you have completed one arm, repeat techniques #57 through #65 on the other arm.

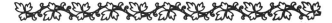

SHOULDERS & NECK

67) ALTERNATING SHOULDER SLIDE

Purpose: This technique helps to release stored shoulder tension.

Positioning: Sit, Japanese style, at the receiver's head.

Procedure: Slowly push one shoulder down toward the receiver's feet. Cup your full hand over the shoulder. Alternate the slow, pushing motion from one shoulder to the other. You must push slowly so that the upper trapezius muscle relaxes. If you shove the shoulder, you will create tension, which is exactly what you do not want to accomplish.

Repetition: Slide each shoulder down toward the feet three times.

Time: 10 seconds.

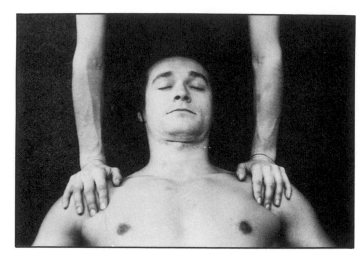

Procedure: Cup both shoulders with your hands, then slowly push the shoulders down toward the receiver's feet. Push both shoulders together.

Repetition: Once is sufficient.

Time: 5 seconds.

69) UPPER TRAPEZIUS BELLY SHOULDER MASSAGE

Purpose: This massage releases tension from the upper trapezius, the major shoulder muscle.

Positioning: Sit, Japanese style, at the receiver's head.

Procedure: Place your fingers under the shoulders and your thumbs on top of the belly of the upper trapezius. Massage and squeeze the entire area. As you do so, incorporate a slight twisting motion. Do not squeeze or massage too hard, for many people will find it too painful. Determine the receiver's tolerance for pain by watching for facial reactions. When you see the receiver begin to grimace, you know you are applying too much force.

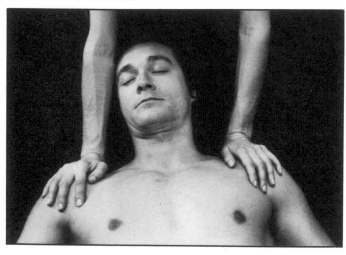

68) SIMULTANEOUS SHOULDER SLIDE

Purpose: This procedure returns both shoulders to their fully relaxed position, releases tension from the shoulder muscles and prepares the shoulders for their position in the next technique, the Upper Trapezius Belly Massage.

Positioning: Sit, Japanese style, at the receiver's head.

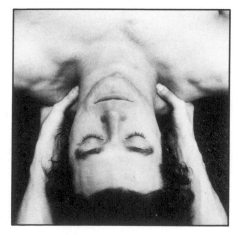

Repetition: Massage the area thoroughly by using approximately twenty-five complete massaging, squeezing and twisting motions. This area needs a lot of manipulation. You will repeat this technique later, after the effects of this manipulation have settled in. When you return to it, you will notice that the area feels looser and less tense, since the previous massaging has released much of the tension from the shoulders.
Time: 30 seconds.

70) SIMULTANEOUS SHOULDER SLIDE

Purpose: Repeat Technique #68. The shoulders tend to rise up from their stretched and relaxed position while you are massaging them. This repetition of the Simultaneous Shoulder Slide returns them to their relaxed position and prepares them for the next technique, Upper Trapezius Thumb Pressure.

71) UPPER TRAPEZIUS THUMB PRESSURE

Purpose: This technique applies firm thumb pressure to the entire length of the shoulders in order to release their tension.
Positioning: Sit, Japanese style, at the receiver's head.
Procedure: Begin applying pressure to the outside edge of the shoulders between the clavicle and spine of the scapula. You will feel a little val-

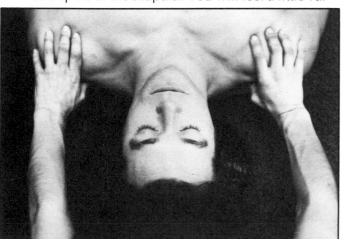

ley with your thumbs, and this is where you begin applying pressure. Move one thumb space at a time as you apply a firm pressure from the outside edge of the shoulders, then along the top of the shoulders and all the way to the neck. Do not skip any area.
Repetition: Apply firm pressure for 3-5 seconds to each area once.
Time: 20 seconds.

72) UPPER THORACIC MASSAGE

Purpose: This technique releases tension from the scapula and shoulder area. Stimulation of the lungs, thyroid and stomach is also accomplished by massaging both sides of the upper thoracic vertebrae.
Positioning: Sit, Japanese style, at the receiver's head.

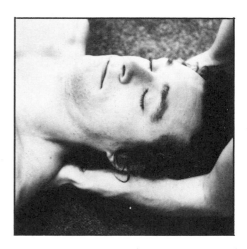

Procedure: Insert the hands, palms up, under the back on either side of the spine. Massage and apply pressure to the back so that it lifts slightly off the mat in a rocking motion. Slide your hands gradually up the length of the spine, massaging alongside the vertebrae, until you reach the base of the neck.
Repetition: Do it five times.
Time: 40 seconds.

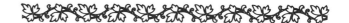

73) UPPER TRAPEZIUS BELLY MASSAGE SHOULDER MASSAGE

Purpose: Repeat Technique #69. Because the shoulders are one of the tensest parts of the body, most people feel neither emotionally nor physically satisfied by only one massage of the belly of the upper trapezius. Repetition of this technique will indicate to you that, although much of the receiver's stored tension has been released, more remains. The repetition will indicate to the receiver your awareness of this lingering pocket of tension, as well as your desire and determination to alleviate it. During this repetition of Technique #69, the receiver usually releases most of the remaining stored shoulder tension. If tense shoulders are a chronic problem with the receiver, repeat Technique #69 again at a later time in the massage.

74) SCAPULA STRETCH

Purpose: The rhomboids muscle originates along the upper thoracic vertebrae and inserts along the vertebral edge of the scapula or shoulder blade. When this muscle is tense, it pulls the scapula out of its proper position. By hooking your fingers along the inside edge of both scapulae and then pulling out and away from the spine, you can help this muscle to relax. You thus help the shoulder blades return to their normal position. This technique will also improve tense shoulders.

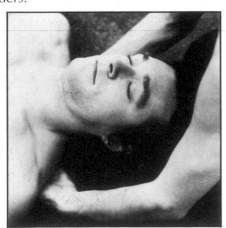

Positioning: Sit, Japanese style, at the receiver's head. Lower your torso sufficiently to execute the technique, but keep your spine erect.
Procedure: Insert both hands, palms up, under the upper back. Hook all four fingers of each hand around the edge of the scapula closest to the spine, then slowly, but firmly pull the scapula out and away from the body.
Repetition: Repeat the pulling motion three times.
Time: 10 seconds.

75) SIMULTANEOUS SHOULDER SLIDE

Purpose: Repeat Technique #68. The execution of Technique #74 tends to cause the shoulders to lose the natural downward position you have helped them to attain. Repetition of the Simultaneous Shoulder Slide returns the shoulders to a relaxed position. It also reminds the receiver where the shoulders should be.

76) SCAPULAE MASSAGE

Purpose: The Scapulae Massage helps to loosen tense shoulders and tense scapulae. It also helps to improve the functioning of the small intestine.
Positioning: Sit, Japanese style, at receiver's head. Lower your torso sufficiently to perform the technique.

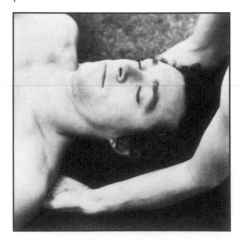

Procedure: Massage the entire surface and edges of the scapulae with four fingers. You need not apply a great deal of pressure because the weight of the receiver's back falling onto your probing fingers will supply sufficient penetration. Use a circular finger massage followed by an inwardly penetrating four-finger pressure to complete the manipulation of each area of the scapulae.

Repetition: Massage each area of the scapulae, then follow with four-finger pressure two or three times.

Time: 20 seconds.

77) NECK STROKING

Purpose: This stroking indicates to the receiver that you are about to begin massaging the neck. As it is incredibly relaxing and pleasurable, many people prefer this simple technique above all others. When correctly executed, it gives the receiver a light-headed sensation and tingling scalp, as well as the feeling that tingles are running up and down the neck, shoulders and spine. Sometimes the tingling will travel all the way to the toes. I interpret these tingles as nerve impulses darting from the cervical region over the entire body because of energy freed and emitted from the neck, a critical point of blockage in the body. These tingles greatly help the body to release much of its stored tension.

Positioning: Sit, Japanese style, at the receiver's head.

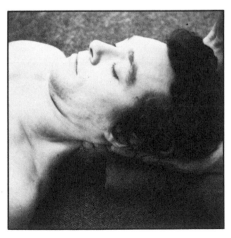

Procedure: Position one hand under the base of the skull and the other under the remainder of the neck. With your hands moving in alternation, employ a pulling motion up from the base of the neck to the back of the skull. Your hands must conform to the contours of the receiver's neck while they are alternately maintaining a good firm grip on the neck and executing an upward pulling motion.

Repetition: Pull hands upward in the Neck Stroking technique at least a total of ten times.

Time: 15 seconds.

78) NECK MASSAGE

Purpose: This technique helps to loosen and relax tense neck muscles.

Positioning: Sit, Japanese style, at the receiver's head.

Procedure: Place one hand, palm down, over the receiver's forehead and the other, palm up, under the neck. Use the fingers and thumb of the hand under the neck to massage and apply pressure to both sides of the entire neck. Reverse hands and repeat. The hand over the forehead remains still.

Repetition: Massage ten times with each hand.

Time: 20 seconds (10 times each hand).

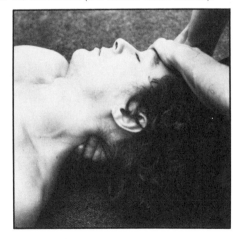

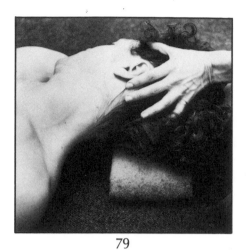
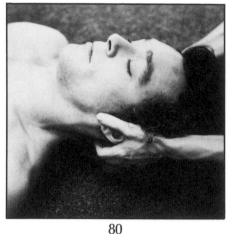
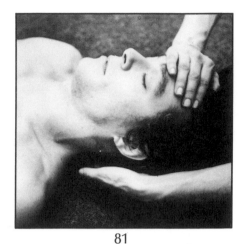

79   80   81

79) HEAD ROLL

Purpose: In addition to relaxing the muscles of the neck and shoulder, this technique helps to release cervical tension.
Positioning: Sit, Japanese style, at the receiver's head.
Procedure: Roll the receiver's head back and forth between your hands. Guide the head to the fullest extent possible in both directions. The receiver must cooperate by allowing the doer to roll the head back and forth freely without any assistance from the receiver. The doer must keep the rolling movement smooth and controlled so that the receiver feels enough trust to let go.
Repetition: Roll head back and forth from right to left a total of five times.
Time: 15 seconds.

80) OUTER PROMINENCES OF THE OCCIPITAL BONE

Purpose: Massaging and applying pressure to the two prominent bulges on either side of the base of the skull releases stored shoulder and neck tension. It is also beneficial to the gall bladder.
Positioning: Sit, Japanese style, at the receiver's head.
Procedure: Place four fingers on each of the prominent bulges at the base of the skull. Alternate a circular massaging motion over and around the prominences with a firm application of four-finger pressure to the prominences. Pressure must be applied slowly. While applying the pressure, lift the head up slightly and pull it back with your fingers. The head will fall back onto the finger tips, and thus provide a firm pressure as well as a slight stretch of the neck.
Repetition: Alternate three circular massages with one firm application of four-finger pressure a total of three times.
Time: 15 seconds.

81) HOLLOW AT BASE OF SKULL GOVERNING 15-16

Purpose: Massaging and applying pressure to these points helps to relieve neck tension. It is also beneficial to the entire nervous system.
Positioning: Sit, Japanese style, at the receiver's head.
Procedure: Place one hand, palm down, on the receiver's forehead. Use the fingers of the other hand, first to massage and then to apply a firm penetrating pressure to the hollow at the base of the skull. Alternate between these two techniques.
Repetition: When massaging, use a circular motion with three fingers. After completing five circular massages apply a firm penetrating pressure with the same three fingers for 3 seconds. Alternate between massaging and firm pressure a total of three times.
Time: 25 seconds.

82) CERVICAL THUMB PRESSURE FOR NECK TENSION

Purpose: This technique relieves neck tension.
Positioning: Sit, Japanese style, at the receiver's head.
Procedure: Turn the receiver's head to one side and place one hand over the forehead. This hand remains still. With the thumb of your other hand, apply pressure along the side of the vertebrae where the nerves emerge from the spinal column. Begin as close to the base of the skull as possible, and work your way down the cervical vertebrae of the neck. Use a medium pressure. Although firm pressure does the job very well, it is usually too painful. Medium pressure will cause the receiver to feel some pain, but it will be interpreted as good pain and will be tolerated by the receiver because its effects will be felt to be beneficial. When you have completed one side of the neck, turn the head and apply pressure to the opposite side. Switch hands.
Repetition: Apply pressure six times down each side of the cervical vertebrae. Hold each pressure application for 7-10 seconds. Do not repeat this technique as once is usually enough.
Time: 60 seconds for each side of the neck or a total of 2 minutes.

83) NECK STRETCH

Purpose: This technique stretches and relaxes the muscles of the neck.
Positioning: Sit, Japanese style, at the receiver's head.
Procedure: Grasp the head with both hands. Lift it straight up so that the receiver's chin touches the clavicle bones, which are the two bony protrusions at the base of the neck on the front of the body. Repeat the lift, but this time direct the head and chin toward the right and then the left shoulder.
Repetition: Stretch twice in each direction.
Time: 15 seconds.

84) HEAD & NECK PULL

Purpose: This technique relaxes the neck and helps to release tension.
Positioning: Sit, Japanese style, at the receiver's head.
Procedure: Place both hands, palms up, under the base of the skull so that your thumbs are below the ears. Grasp the head firmly and pull it toward you.
Repetition: Repeat twice.
Time: 5 seconds.

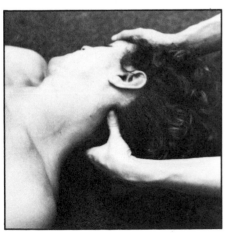

82

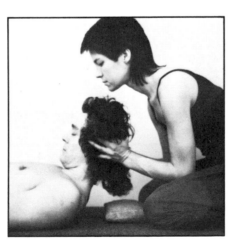

83

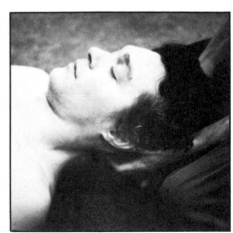

84

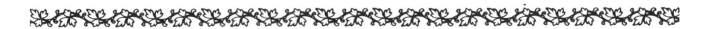

85) NECK SEA WAVES

Purpose: This final technique performed on the neck is another of those particularly marvelous ones. At the same time that it relaxes and releases stress, it provides the sensation to the receiver that her/his head and neck is floating and bobbing on a sea of waves. Everyone loves it.

Positioning: Sit, Japanese style, at the receiver's head.

Procedure: Place both hands, palms up, under the neck. Pull the neck up with both hands and let the head roll freely along with your motions. Trace an imaginary circle in the air while holding the neck. The circle should move in a direction from the receiver toward the doer. The neck is raised off the mat at the highest point of the imaginary circle and touches the mat at the lowest.

Repetition: Make ten circles.

Time: 15 seconds.

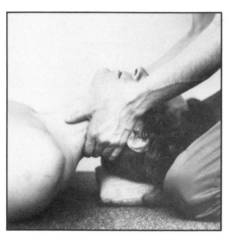

HEAD & EARS

86) FINGER SCRATCH SCALP

Purpose: This technique feels GREAT! It is one of the most popular. The Finger Scratch improves circulation to the scalp, face, eyes and sinuses. It improves, too, the condition of the hair. If employed faithfully several times a day, this technique can also often prompt growth of new hair.

Positioning: Sit, Japanese style, at the receiver's head.

Procedure: Use the tips of your fingers, not your nails. Position your fingers and thumbs behind and to either side of the ears. Using a back-and-forth pulling and sliding motion, scratch the entire scalp. Keep your fingers fairly rigid, and frequently change the direction of your pulling and sliding motion to stimulate the scalp more effectively.

Repetition: Cover each area of the scalp more than once. Keep the scratching motion on the slow side. Although a fast scratch feels good, it will not sustain the receiver's peaceful frame of mind.

Time: 25 seconds.

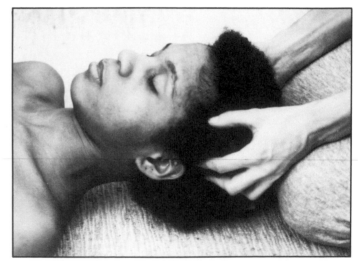

87) GALL BLADDER PRESS

Purpose: This press helps to stimulate and improve gall bladder function. It feels good too.
Positioning: Sit, Japanese style, at the receiver's head.
Procedure: Apply firm pressure to the path of the Gall Bladder Meridian around the ear with your index, third and fourth fingers. See illustration indicating the path the meridian follows around the ear.
Repetition: Repeat twice. Hold each pressure application for 3-5 seconds.
Time: 10 seconds.

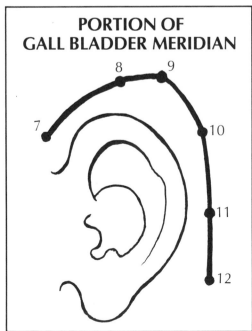

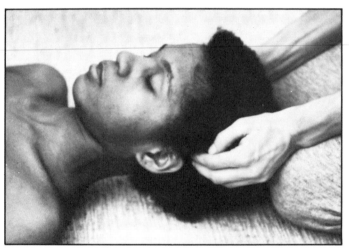

**PORTION OF
GALL BLADDER MERIDIAN**

88) SINUS PRESS

Purpose: This technique relieves congestion and other sinus afflictions.
Positioning: Sit, Japanese style, at the receiver's head.
Procedure: Apply firm thumb pressure from the widow's peak, which is the center of the hairline on the forehead, back along an imaginary center line to the point where the skull drops back. Pressure cannot successfully be applied to the back of the skull from this position.
Repetition: Repeat twice.
Time: 20 seconds.

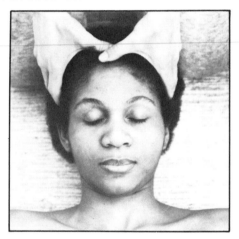

89) FINGER SCRATCH SCALP

Purpose: Repeat Technique #86.

90) GENERAL EAR STIMULATION

Purpose: Stimulation of the entire ear prepares the receiver for the ear massage.
Positioning: Sit, Japanese style, at the receiver's head.
Procedure: Place your index and third fingers on either side of the the receiver's ears. Use a back-and-forth motion and make plenty of contact with the ear.
Repetition: Slide the fingers back and forth a total of five times.
Time: 10 seconds.

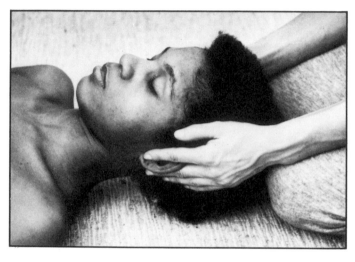

91) EAR MASSAGE

See diagram of Auricular Reflex Points
Purpose: This technique feels marvelous. It also stimulates the reflex points of the ear. Auricular therapy has been practiced in France for many years. Dr. Bordes was the first physician to establish a correlation between auricular reflex points and sciatic nerve problems. Noting that many of his patients with such problems had a scar on the same auricular reflex point, he investigated further and discovered that their local blacksmith had burned the ear at that particular point to relieve their pain.

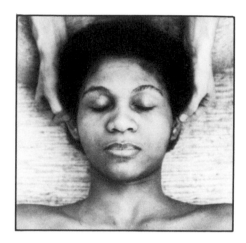

Positioning: Sit, Japanese style, at the receiver's head.
Procedure: Use your fingers and thumbs to massage the entire ear. Do not focus on any one part, but rather massage and manipulate the entire ear.
Repetition: Massage the entire ear twice.
Time: 30 seconds.

92) EAR LOBE PRESSURE

Purpose: Pressure to the ear lobe benefits the face, eyes, sinus and ears.
Positioning: Sit, Japanese style, at the receiver's head.
Procedure: Using your thumbs and index fingers, apply pressure to the entire lobe of the ear.
Repetition: Apply pressure to the entire lobe twice. Hold pressure for 3 seconds.
Time: 10 seconds.

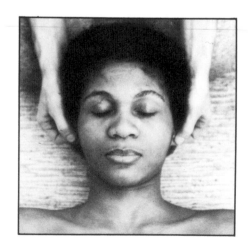

93) MASSAGE & APPLY PRESSURE TO THE EAR

Purpose: This technique is for the further stimulation of ear acupuncture pressure points.
Positioning: Sit, Japanese style, at the receiver's head.
Procedure: Insert your index finger into the eminences and depressions of the ear. Alternate massage and pressure.
Repetition: Repeat twice.
Time: 15 seconds.

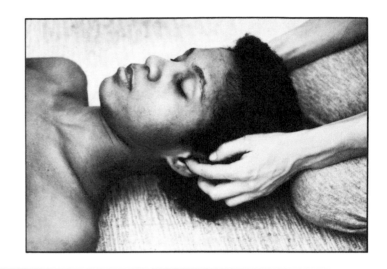

AURICULOTHERAPY

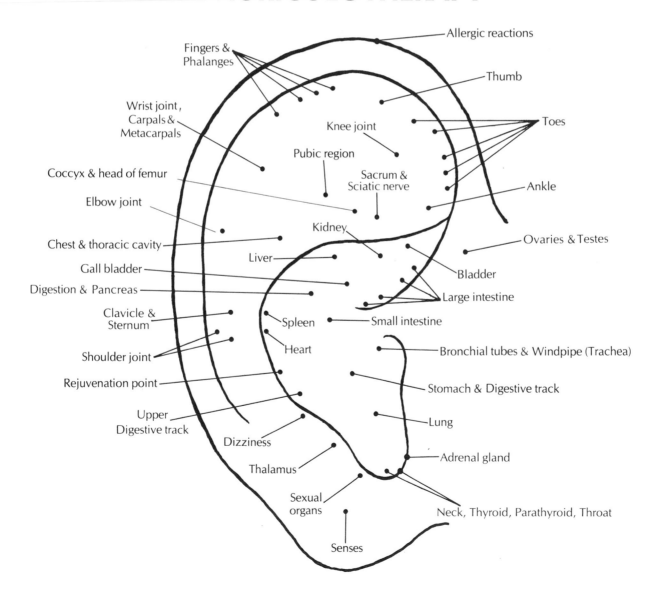

FACE

94) FACE LIFT

Purpose: This technique acts as a greeting to the face. It improves circulation and muscle tone. It also feels really good.
Positioning: Sit, Japanese style, at the receiver's head.
Procedure: Place one hand on either side of the receiver's face. Beginning at the jaw, slide your hands up the face, over the cheekbones and then over the forehead. Allow your hands to conform to the contours of the receiver's face.
Repetition: Repeat twice.
Time: 5 seconds.

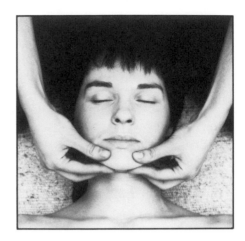

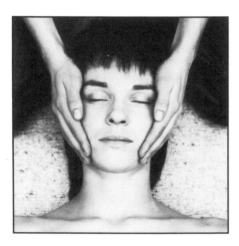

95) CHIN LINE STROKE

Purpose: This technique helps to relax the jaw and trim the chin line.
Positioning: Sit, Japanese style, at the receiver's head.
Procedure: Place your fingers under the chin line and your thumbs above the chin line. Begin at the center of the chin and stroke outward to the jaw. A little oil is helpful for this technique, and the next one too.
Repetition: Repeat three times.
Time: 5 seconds.

96) CHIN LINE FIRMER

Purpose: This technique helps reduce double or triple chins.
Positioning: Sit, Japanese style, at the receiver's head.
Procedure: Use your middle fingers to stroke under the receiver's chin. Alternate your right with your left hand as you execute the stroking.
Repetition: Stroke each side of the chin under the jaw five times. Repeat more often if the receiver has a double chin.
Time: 10 seconds.

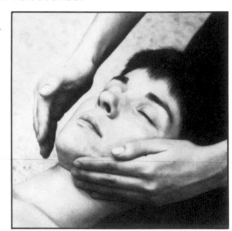

97) GUM PRESSURE

Purpose: This technique helps to improve the circulation to the gums and nerves of the teeth. It also helps firm the lip line.

Positioning: Sit, Japanese style, at the receiver's head.

Procedure: Apply gentle pressure through the skin to the gums of the lower and upper jaw. Use a four-finger pressure technique. Do not press too firmly, for the tissue is sensitive here.

Repetition: One application of pressure to each area of the gums is sufficient.

Time: 5 seconds.

98) MANDIBLE MASSAGE

Purpose: Many people store tension in the muscles of the jaw. This technique helps to release it.

Positioning: Sit, Japanese style, at the receiver's head.

Procedure: Use a circular massaging motion with three fingers over the joints of the jaw. Next, apply a fairly firm pressure for 3 seconds, but be sensitive with your pressure as this is very often a sore spot. Watch the receiver's face for signs of discomfort.

Repetition: Repeat two or three times. Be sure, however, that you have thoroughly massaged the muscles around and over the flexible portion of the jaw, prior to applying firm pressure to the tempromandibular joint.

Time: 30 seconds.

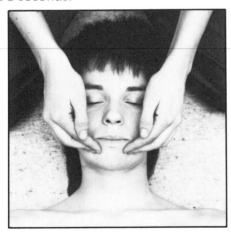

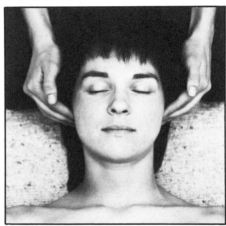

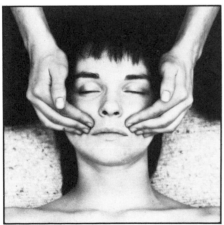

99) CHEEKBONE PRESSURE FOR SINUS PROBLEMS

Purpose: Pressure applied to the cheekbones helps to relieve stuffy sinuses.
Positioning: Sit, Japanese style, at the receiver's head.
Procedure: Use three fingers on the lower part of the cheekbone and your thumbs on the upper part. Apply a firm pressure.
Repetition: Repeat several times if the receiver has chronic or acute sinus problems.
Time: 15 seconds.

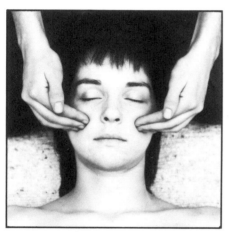

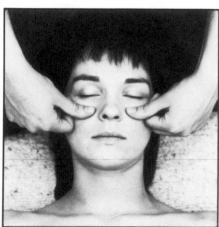

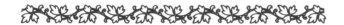

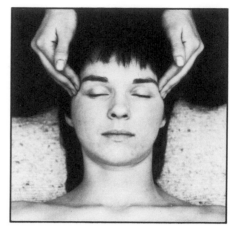

100) TEMPLE MASSAGE

Purpose: This technique is very relaxing and calming. It helps to release facial tension and benefits the eyes.
Positioning: Sit, Japanese style, at the receiver's head.
Procedure: Use three fingers to massage the temples. Begin with a fairly light, circular massaging motion and gradually increase the pressure. Use the pads of your fingers, not your finger tips.
Repetition: Complete ten circular massaging motions.
Time: 10 seconds.

101) FOREHEAD SLIDE

Purpose: Not only does this technique help to relax the muscles of the forehead, but it also helps to discourage vertical and horizontal wrinkles.
Positioning: Sit, Japanese style, at the receiver's head.
Procedure: Position your thumbs between the eyebrows. Slide your thumbs out along the forehead to the hairline just above the ear. Place your thumbs slightly above their previous position between the eyebrows, and then repeat the technique. Continue in this fashion until the entire forehead has been relaxed. Next, use your four fingers to relax the forehead in an upward direction. Begin by placing the fingers of both hands directly above the eyebrows. Gently slide the fingers over the skin until you reach the hairline.
Repetition: The first part of this technique need be done only once. The vertical slide from the eyebrows to the hairline should be repeated two or three times.
Time: 20 seconds.

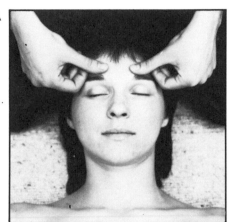

101 A

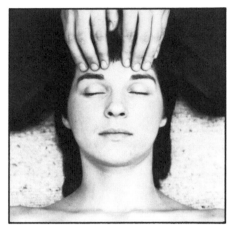

101 B

102) ORBIT OF THE EYE PRESSURE FOR SINUS & EYESTRAIN

Purpose: Pressure applied to the orbits of the eyes will improve sinus conditions and decrease eye-strain. Any condition of the eyes will benefit from this technique.

Positioning: Sit, Japanese style, at the receiver's head.

Procedure: Apply pressure to the upper part of the orbits of the eyes with all four fingers. Thumb pressure is more suitable for the lower orbits. Do not be heavy-handed. These points are often tender.

Repetition: Two pressure applications suffice the upper orbits. Apply pressure to the lower orbits as you move from the inner corner to the outer and hold each application for 3-5 seconds. One application of thumb pressure to each area of the lower orbits is sufficient.

Time: 20 seconds.

103) EYEBALL PRESSURE

Purpose: Pressure here relaxes and strengthens the eyes.

Positioning: Sit, Japanese style, at the receiver's head.

Procedure: Rest all four fingers over the eyeballs and cheekbones. Apply a light to medium pressure. Release the pressure, then slowly slide fingers off the eyes and cheekbones.

Repetition: Unnecessary.

Time: 10 seconds.

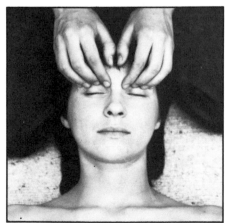

102 A

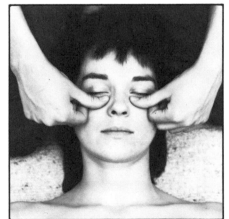

102 B

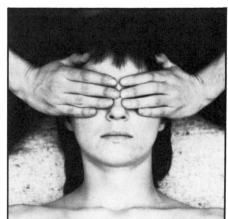

103

CHAPTER V

Massage—Special Applications

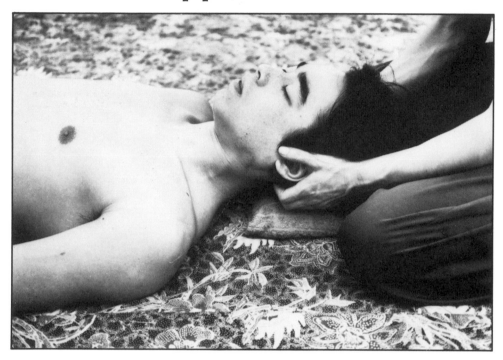

1) "QUICKIE" MASSAGE TECHNIQUES

A Quickie Massage is a wonderful experience. In a minimum of time and with little preparation you can completely change the way your partner or friend feels. Exhaustion, tired eyes, aching back, sore feet, heavy limbs and lack of enthusiasm can be massaged away in a short period of fifteen to twenty-five minutes and can be replaced with renewed energy and freedom from aches and pains due to overwork or worry. An evening or day that might have been spent feeling exhausted, pained and miserable can quickly become a time for fun and new adventures.

Below you will find some helpful suggestions and reminders to make your Quickie Massage a complete success. ENJOY!

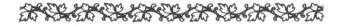

- Execute techniques slowly and with great compassion. Quickie Massage does not mean that the techniques are to be executed quickly

- NEVER apply pressure suddenly. Gradual penetration is always the rule

- Try to be conscious of your posture as you massage

- NEVER apply pressure directly to the spinal column

- When twisting, pulling, stretching or flexing any part of the body, always proceed SLOWLY

- Spread a sheet on the floor, dim the lights, silence the phone and begin. Lengthy preparations are unnecessary

Some of the techniques for the Quickie Massage have been extracted from the Complete 60-Minute Body Massage in Chapter IV. Others will be new to you. Those techniques that have already been discussed in the Complete 60-Minute Body Massage are once again illustrated with photographs so that you won't continually have to turn back the pages to refer to the previous section. In the event of any confusion as to what to do or why you are doing it, refer to the more detailed description of the technique in Chapter IV.

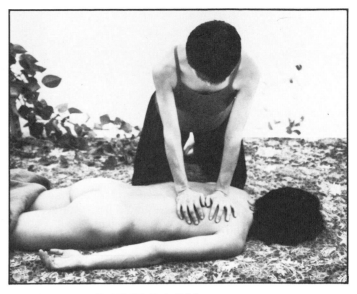

ROCKING THE BACK

This technique prepares the back for deeper penetration and relaxes the muscles near the spine. Sit, Japanese style, perpendicular to the receiver's spine. Use the heels of your hands to rock the back. Rock the upper, middle and lower back five times each. Total time: 60 seconds.

DEEP BREATHING TECHNIQUE

Place the heels of your hands on either side of the upper back. Instruct the receiver to inhale and then exhale. On the exhale, slowly apply a firm, gradually increasing pressure into the back. When you reach the bottom of the rib cage, change the orientation of your hands so that they are perpendicular to the spine and use less pressure so as not to break the floating ribs. The last application of pressure will be directly over the sacrum. Total time: 60 seconds.

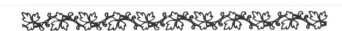

SPINE TRACING

Spine tracing releases superfical spinal tension, relaxes the receiver and prepares the back for the more intense techniques which follow. Sit, Japanese style, next to the receiver. Place three fingers on either side of the spine, then very slowly begin to pull your fingers down the sides of the spinal column. Continue to the tip of the coccyx. Repeat two times. Total time: 20 seconds.

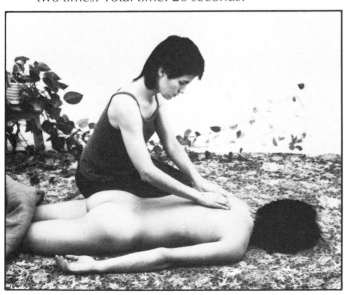

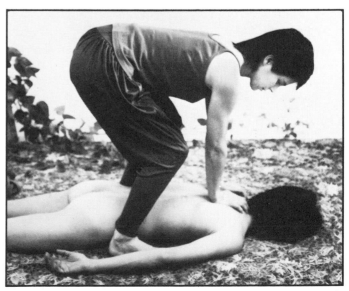

VERTEBRAE TECHNIQUE

Sit at the receiver's side so that you are parallel to the spine, or else straddle the receiver on your knees. In the case of a large person, straddle the body on your feet with your knees bent. Massage 3-5 seconds along side each pair of vertebrae to prepare the receiver for penetration. Penetrate for 5 seconds, then massage 3-5 seconds to soothe. The massaging and penetration should be performed with your thumbs. Place them on either side of the spine close to the vertebrae. Begin midway between the scapula and work your way down the spine to the sacrum.
Total time: 3-5 minutes.

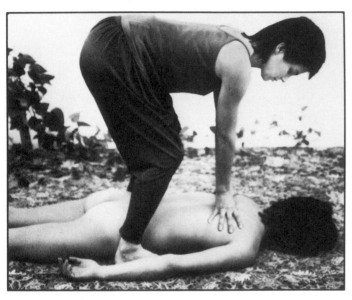

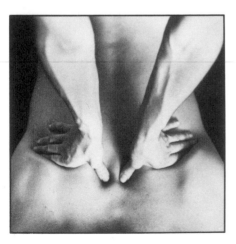

UPPER TRAPEZIUS SHOULDER MASSAGE

Massage, knead and squeeze the muscles between the shoulders and the neck. Use your fingers to loosen and relax the muscles. Follow with firm thumb pressure to any part of the muscle that feels tense or knotted. Total time: 30 seconds.

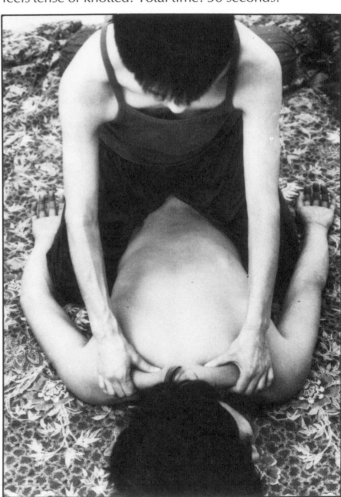

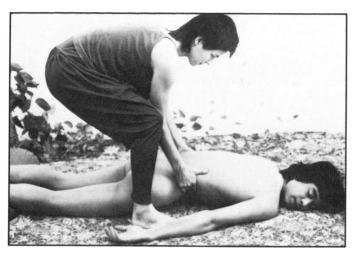

WAIST LIFT

Slide your hands under the receiver's waist and pull the flesh or the entire trunk up off the mat. Apply pressure into the waist as you lift upward. Repeat three times. Total time: 10 seconds.

LATISSIMUS DORSI MASSAGE

Thoroughly massage the fullest part of the muscle by grabbing it in your hands, then knead, twist and release it. Repeat about ten times. As this muscle corresponds to the pancreas, which controls the blood sugar metabolism, massaging it during or immediately after meals aids in digestion. Total time: 10 seconds.

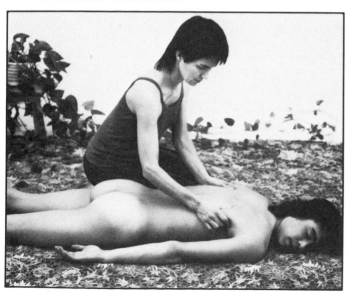

UPPER TRAPEZIUS SHOULDER MASSAGE

Repeat this technique as described previously for an additional 30 seconds.

ARM PRESSURE

With the heels of your hands, simultaneously apply a firm, but sensitive pressure from the top of the arms to the wrists. Use three pressure applications on both the upper arms and forearms. Encourage the arms to roll with each application of pressure.
Total time: 30 seconds.

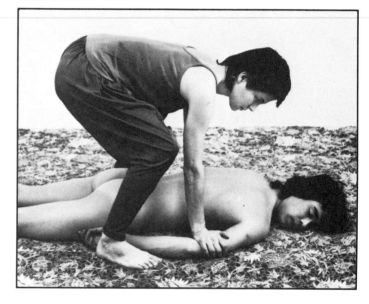

ARM & FINGER STRETCH

Grasp the forearms above the wrists. <u>Slowly</u> pull the arms until the shoulders rise off the mat, then release. Next, massage, twist and pull each pair of fingers simultaneously. Begin with the little fingers and move toward the thumbs. Don't be rough. Pull and twist slowly, compassionately. This technique loosens the joints of the upper appendages and affects all the meridians of the arms which include the Heart, Circulation/Sex, Lungs, Large Intestines, Small Intestine and Triple Warmer. Total time: 30 seconds.

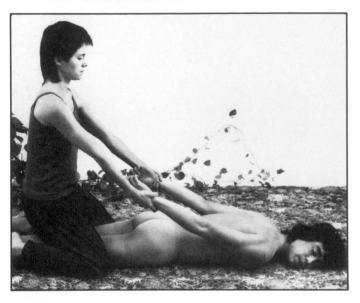

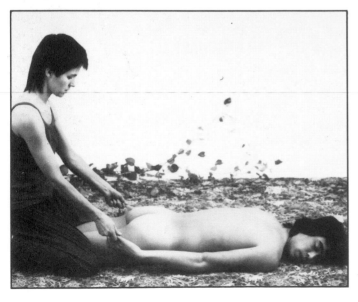

SHOULDER LIFT

Slide your hands under the shoulders. Instruct the receiver not to help but to remain limp, like a rag doll. Slowly begin to lift the shoulders, and then the upper trunk, off the mat. Do not lift suddenly or too high. The photograph indicates how high you should lift the trunk. This technique broadens the chest, relaxes the shoulders and flexes the spine. Total time: 5-10 seconds.

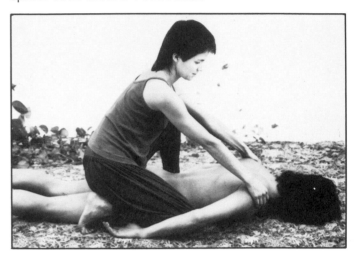

KNEADING THE BUTTOCKS

Knead the buttocks with the heels of your hands. This technique benefits general circulation, the sciatic nerve and the gluteus muscles, which are related to the sexual and reproductive organs. Straddle the receiver's legs and apply a firm kneading pressure. Total time: 20 seconds.

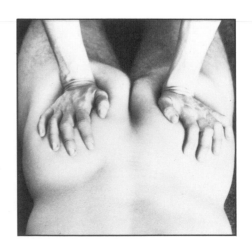

THIGH & LEG BLADDER MERIDIAN

Apply firm pressure for 3-5 seconds with the heel of your hand down the center of the back of the thigh and leg. As the crease of the knee is a very sensitive area of the leg, apply only a very light pressure here. Many people also have tender calf muscles, although they are not usually as tender as the back of the knee. Use less pressure over the calf than over the thigh, but slightly more than that used for the crease of the knee. This technique affects the Bladder Meridian and its associated functions. It also relaxes and releases tension from the leg. Apply pressure to the thigh four times and to the leg four times.
Total time: 30 seconds.

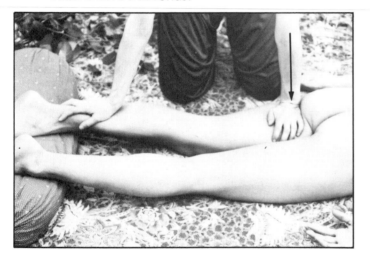

KNEE FLEX

Grasp the feet, bend the legs and *gently* rock them back and forth five times. Next, allow the legs to fall to the side as much as they are able. Rock them in this position five more times. This technique loosens the knee joints and stretches the quadriceps in the front of the thighs. Don't rock vigorously or with too much pressure.
Total time: 10-15 seconds.

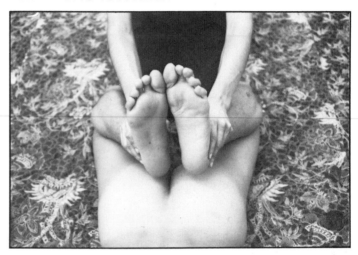

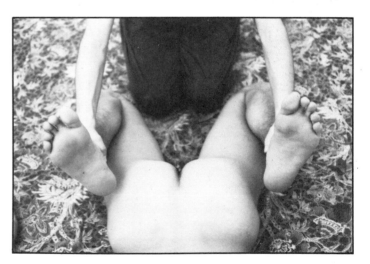

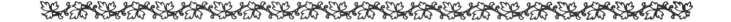

FOOT WALK

With your back turned to the receiver's back, stand on the receiver's feet with your heels. Shift your weight back and forth from one foot to the other. Shift your weight slowly and allow it to gradually bear down on the feet. Beware of the arch of the receiver's foot, as too much pressure on the arch can be painful and could snap the metatarsal bone located directly above the big toe. Before you begin this technique, instruct the receiver to inform you <u>immediately</u> if the pressure is too great. The remainder of the foot can safely tolerate most of your weight for a few seconds. Try to apply pressure to the entire bottom of each foot. Keep in mind the foot diagram and the organs that are affected. Total time: 60 seconds.

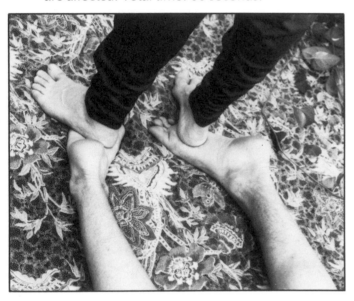

SPINAL SWING

Grasp the feet and *slowly* lift the pelvis off the mat. *Very gently* and *slowly* swing the legs from side to side a total of five times in each direction. Do not lift the thighs more than two or three inches off the mat. This technique increases spinal flexibility. Total time: 10-15 seconds. Do not use this technique if the receiver suffers from extreme low back pain.

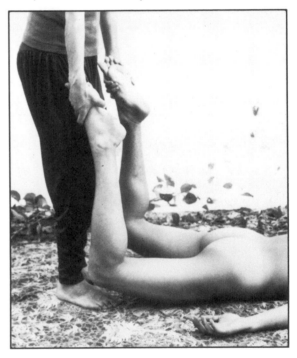

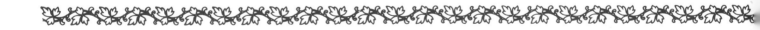

FOOT & TOE ACKNOWLEDGMENT

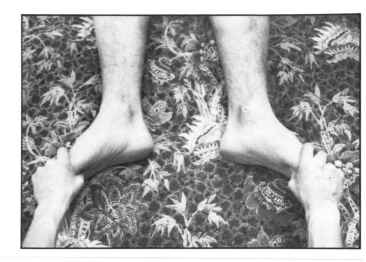

Because this is a quickie massage and because you have already walked on the receiver's feet, it is not necessary to devote as much time to the feet as you would during a full body massage. Acknowledgment is sufficient to get the blood flowing back to the heart and to stimulate the nerves and internal organs. Squeeze, massage and twist each toe, then apply firm thumb pressure to the arch of the foot and superficially acknowledge the bottom of each foot with your thumb. Complete the foot work with a technique called rolling, i.e. grasp one foot with both hands and twist it in opposite directions from the toes to the ankle. Do not to burn the skin as you twist. Total time: 2 minutes (1 minute for each foot).

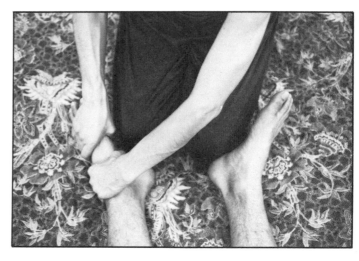

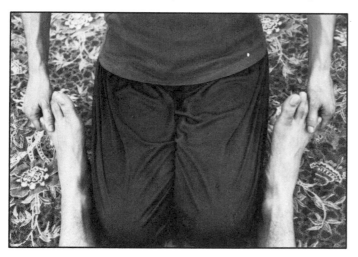

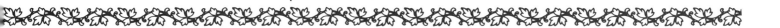

LEG TWIST

Apply pressure to the sides of both feet, first by pressing them outward and then by pushing them in toward the center of the body. This technique loosens the ankle, knee and hip joints. It also feels very good. Push five times each direction. Total time: 10 seconds.

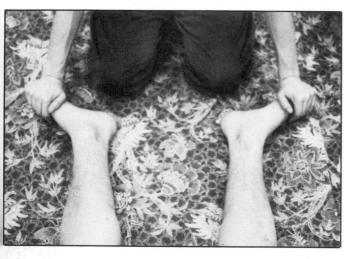

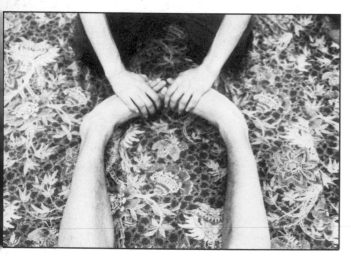

LEG FLEX & ROTATION

Bend the leg at the knee and slowly rotate the leg four times each direction. Encourage the receiver to completely relax so that you can perform the rotations without the receiver's anticipation or assistance. This loosens the joints of the leg. Repeat on the other leg. Total time: 20 seconds.

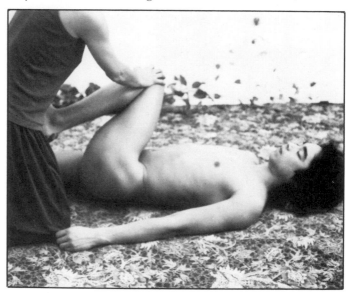

SACRAL PRESSURE

Bend the receiver's legs at the knees. Position the thighs perpendicular to the mat. Cup the knees with your hands and allow some of your body weight to rest directly on top of the knees. Release your weight slowly. Do not apply sudden pressure, as this will not feel good to the receiver. This technique feels wonderful and helps to release lower back tension. Total time: 10 seconds.

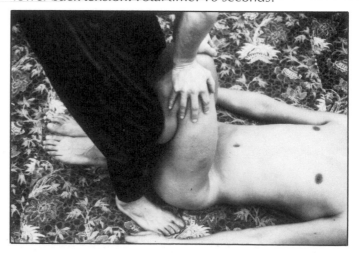

WAIST LIFT

Insert your hands under the receiver's waist and lift up the flesh or lift the trunk off the mat. This technique feels wonderful and stimulates the liver and gall bladder functions. Repeat three times. Total time: 10 seconds.

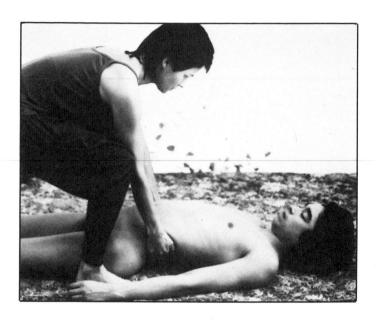

ABDOMINAL MASSAGE

Begin a circular, sweeping motion on the lower right side of the abdomen. Continue upward, across the top of the abdomen and then down the left side. Alternate hands as you sweep around the abdomen. Repeat three times.
Total time: 10 seconds.

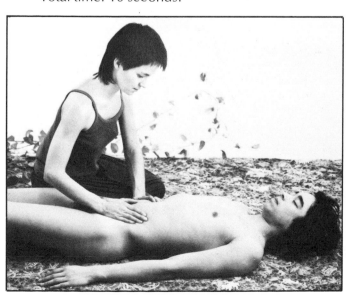

RIB LYMPHATIC FLUSH

Slide your fingers along between the ribs from the side of the torso up to the sternum. Repeat as many times as necessary to insure that most of the intercostal spaces between the ribs have been reached at least twice. This technique feels wonderful and releases stagnant lymph fluid.
Total time: 30 seconds.

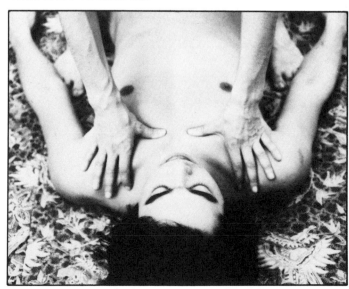

CHEST LYMPHATIC RELEASE

With your thumbs, massage between the ribs on either side of the sternum. Begin under the clavicle protuberances and continue down to the bottom of the breasts or below the pectoralis muscles. This technique benefits the kidneys, heart, thyroid, lungs, stomach and gall bladder.
Total time: 40 seconds.

SHOULDER MASSAGE

Insert your hands, palms up, under the upper trapezius muscles. Massage the fullest part of the muscles with your fingers and thumbs. Neck and shoulder tension is released with this technique. Total time: 30 seconds.

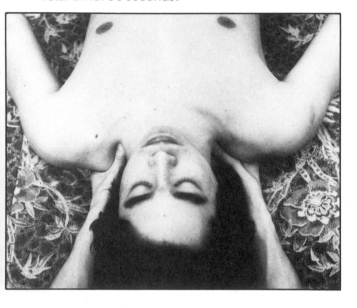

NECK MASSAGE

Hold the receiver's head to one side in one hand and insert your other hand, palm up, under the neck. Massage the nape of the neck with your fingers and thumb. Switch hands and repeat on the opposite side. This technique helps to release neck tension. Total time: 30 seconds.

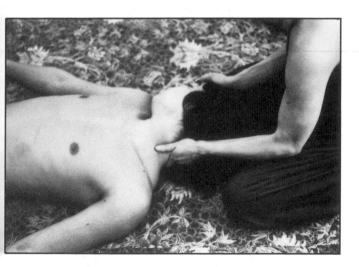

BASE OF THE SKULL MASSAGE

There is a prominent knob on either side of the base of the back of the skull. Position the fingers of each hand over each of the knobs and massage deeply and firmly. This technique releases neck and shoulder tension and stimulates the gall bladder. Total time: 30 seconds.

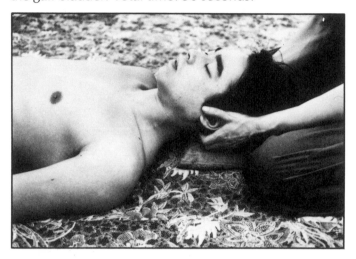

UPPER BACK OR UPPER THORACIC VERTEBRAE TECHNIQUE

Insert your hands, palms up, under the back on either side of the spine. Position your finger tips so that they rest between the shoulder blades, or between the fifth and sixth thoracic vertebrae on either side of the spine. Begin a circular rocking and massaging motion on either side of the vertebrae.

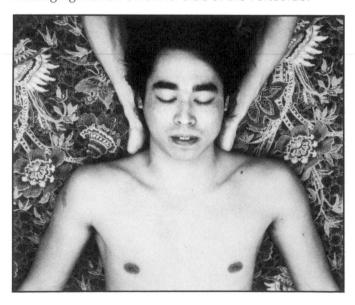

Complete five circular massaging motions, then move up to the fourth and fifth vertebrae and repeat. Continue to the base of the neck. The motion is more difficult to describe than it is to perform. Begin by pushing your finger tips up into the back and then, in a scooping motion toward you, pull your fingers slightly off and back around to same spot. Your finger tips are making a circle that moves toward you and then away from you. At the top of the circle you press your fingers into the receiver's back. Repeat five times between each pair of vertebrae.
Total time: 30 seconds.

SHOULDER BLADE TECHNIQUE

Slide your hands, palms up, under the receiver's shoulder blades. Lift your finger tips up and into the surface of the shoulder blades. Massage each area with circular motions for 3-5 seconds. Then, firmly press your finger tips into the areas you have just massaged and hold the pressure for 3 seconds. Massage and apply pressure to the entire surface of the shoulder blades.
Total time: 60 seconds.

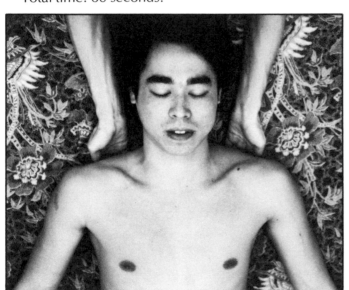

SCALP MASSAGE

Thoroughly massage the entire scalp with your finger tips. Frequently change the direction of your pulling and sliding motions to stimulate the scalp most effectively. Turn the receiver's head to one side when massaging the back of the head, and hold the receiver's forehead with one hand and massage the back of the head with the other. Switch hands and repeat the scalp massage on the other side of the back of the receiver's head. Total time: 30 seconds.

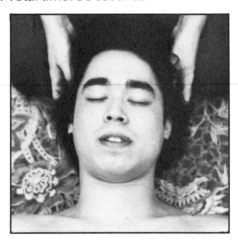

EAR MASSAGE

Use your fingers and thumbs to massage the ears. Go inside as well as behind the ears.
Total time: 30 seconds.

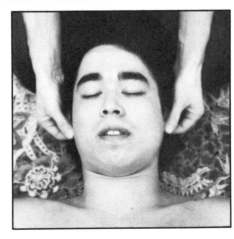

FACE ACKNOWLEDGMENT

There is not enough time to massage the face thoroughly when you are giving a quickie massage. Simply position your hands over the chin and gently slide your hands over the face up into the hairline. The face does not feel neglected as long as it is acknowledged. Repeat five times. Total time: 30 seconds.

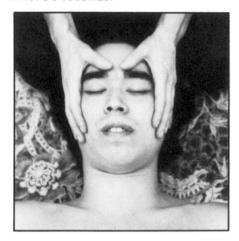

EYE SLIDE

Position your fingers over the receiver's closed eyes and allow them to rest there, very gently, for 20 seconds. Next, very slowly, slide your fingers off the eyes, out over the temples and into the hair line just above the ears. Be careful not to stretch the skin. Total time: 30 seconds.

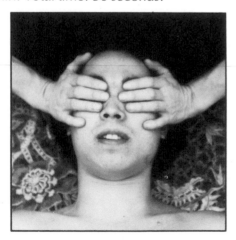

FINISHING TOUCH

Gently rest your finger tips over the eyes and place the palms of your hands over the forehead to make contact with the frontal eminence neurovascular holding points. Remain totally still for approximately 30 seconds while holding your hands in this position. Then, over a period of 20 seconds, very slowly begin to withdraw your hands and fingers from the receiver's eyes and forehead. Once your hands are off the face, continue to withdraw them slowly away from the receiver. A sudden withdrawal is disturbing and tends to startle the receiver, for cool air rushes in where your hands were once providing warmth. Total time: 160 seconds.

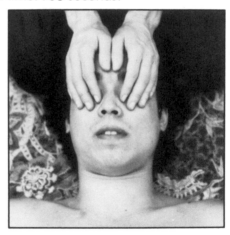

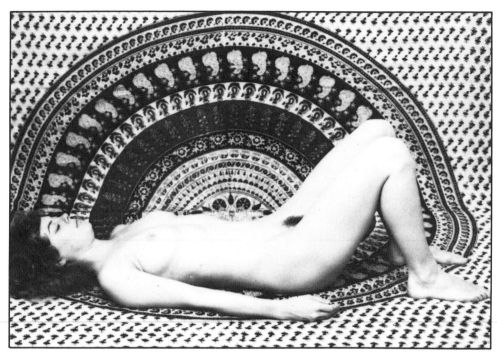

2)HOW TO DO SELF-MASSAGE

Self-massage enables you to care for yourself, both emotionally and physically, on a regular basis. It works, it's simple and it's cheap. No one knows your body better than you. Take advantage of this knowledge by treating yourself to the wonderful sensations and healing powers of self-massage. Granted, massaging yourself is not as fulfilling as being massaged by someone else, but it is much more rewarding, satisfying and effective than most people believe.

People have always touched themselves to relieve pain and release tension. Prehistoric humans no doubt rubbed their abdomens when they were experiencing digestive difficulties and held their foreheads when they were upset or concentrating. Both are extremely common and effective self-massage or self-touch techniques that are utilized on a totally subconscious level of awareness. It's time to acknowledge that our instincts are wise. It is healthy and practical to care for your body and mind. So set aside time once a week, or more often, to improve your health through self-massage.

The method of self-massage taught in this book is unique because it's done exclusively in the reclining position. It thereby eliminates most of the strain and fatigue normally associated with self-massage. The Alexander Rest Position is perfect for self-massage because it minimizes the effort expended. Why fight gravity when it can be used to your advantage?

With legs bent and effortlessly balanced, tilt your pelvis back into the floor (flattening the arch of your lower back) and stretch your entire spine from the coccyx to the base of the skull. Raise your head on a 1"-2" pillow to correct your cervical alignment.

Consider the following while you massage:

* Once you have mastered a technique, focus your concentration more on how the technique feels than on how to implement it

* Keep your body relaxed; don't tense up

* Don't use muscle power; work from your hara

* Close your eyes as you work for greater realization of the different sensations you are evoking from your body

* Try to duplicate the positions shown in the photographs as they will offer you the maximum comfort and greatest result

THE FEET & LEGS

Complete one foot and leg before proceeding to the other.

ANKLE ROTATIONS

Grasp the ball of your foot. Make three slow rotations clockwise, then three counter-clockwise. Feel the stretch and listen for the cracking as the joint loosens up.

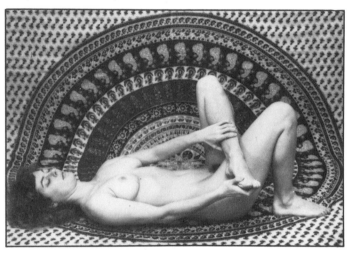

FIVE TOE ROTATIONS

Hold your toes with one hand and stabilize your foot with the other. Rotate all toes three times in each direction.

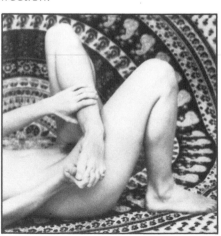

INDIVIDUAL TOE ROTATIONS

Rotate each toe twice in each direction

TOE SQUEEZE

Squeeze and massage each toe from its tip toward the foot. This forces blood back to the heart and out of the toes.

BETWEEN TOE SLIDE

Insert your index finger between each toe. Slide it back and forth three times.

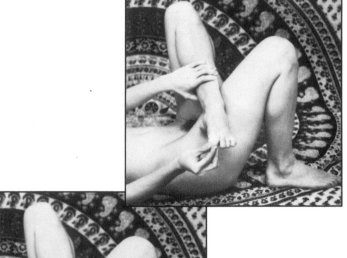

GENERAL SOLE MASSAGE

Use your thumbs to superficially massage the entire bottom of your foot. Circular massaging motions are best to prepare your foot for the more penetrating techniques that follow.

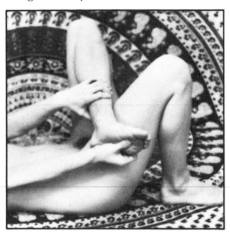

PINCH OUTSIDE EDGE OF FOOT

Use your thumb and index finger to pinch and twist the skin. Begin under the toes and work your way down.

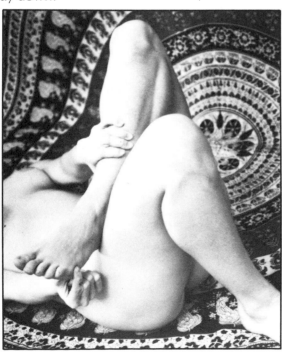

SPINAL COLUMN REFLEX POINTS

Use your thumb or knuckle to apply firm 5-second pressure first to the side of the heel, then up the arch to the top of the big toe.

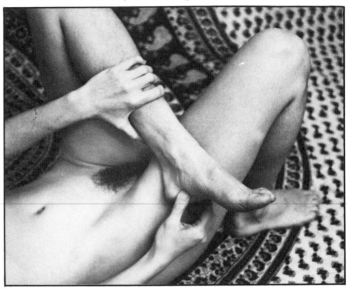

BASE OF THE TOES MASSAGE

Use four fingers to massage the areas under the toes which correspond to the eyes, ears, sinuses and teeth. Press firmly into the bones for 3-5 seconds.

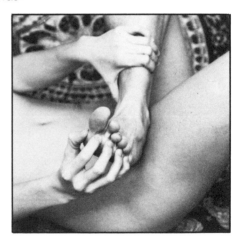

BOTTOMS OF THE FEET REFLEX POINTS

Refer to the foot chart. Apply firm thumb or knuckle pressure to each of the reflex areas for 3-5 seconds. Note that each area corresponds to a particular organ.

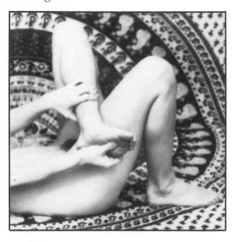

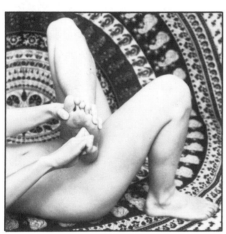

METATARSAL FAN SLIDE

Insert your fingers into the spaces between the metatarsal bones at the base of the toes. Slide your fingers along in the grooves, then up and over the ankle. Repeat three times. This affects the lungs, chest and breast.

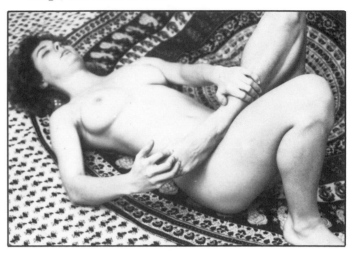

ANKLEBONE MASSAGE

Massage both anklebones of one foot at the same time with your fingers and thumbs. Cup each of the bones with the fingers and thumb of each hand and move them in unison. Use a circular massaging motion. This improves reproductive and sexual organs, hip and sciatic nerve inflamations and back tension.

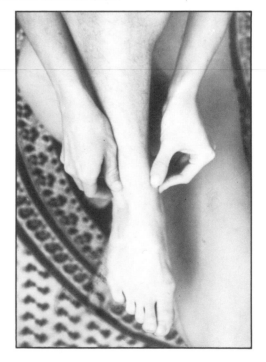

REPRODUCTIVE & SEXUAL ORGANS

Use your thumb and index finger to firmly massage the hollow between the anklebone and heel for 5-10 seconds.

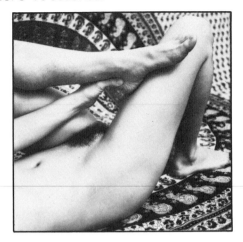

ACHILLES TENDON MASSAGE

Use your thumb and first two fingers to massage and squeeze the Achilles tendon firmly. Sciatic nerve and rectal conditions, as well as disturbances of the reproductive and sexual organs, benefit from frequent utilization of this technique.

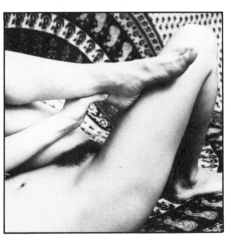

CALF/BLADDER PRESSURE POINTS

Apply a medium to firm pressure to the indicated points with your fingers for 3-5 seconds. Tired legs, bladder problems and sciatic nerve conditions respond to these pressure points.

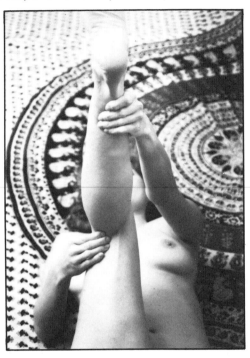

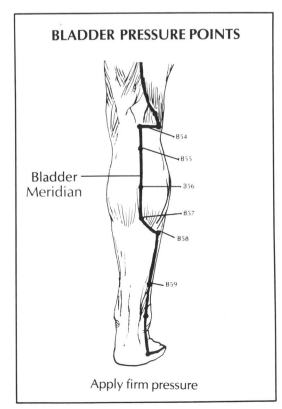

BLADDER PRESSURE POINTS

Bladder
Meridian

B54
B55
356
B57
B58
B59

Apply firm pressure

BACK OF THE THIGH
BLADDER POINTS

Use four fingers to apply a firm penetrating pressure for 3-5 seconds to the bladder points on the back of the thigh. This technique improves bladder conditions and functions.

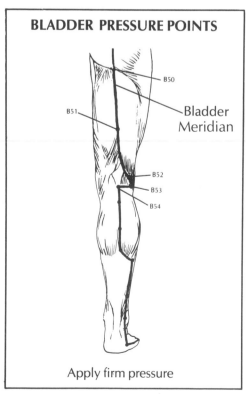

BLADDER PRESSURE POINTS

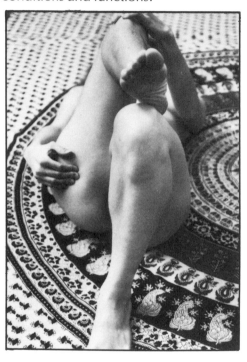

B50

B51

Bladder
Meridian

B52

B53

B54

Apply firm pressure

SMALL INTESTINE
NEURO-LYMPHATIC
MASSAGE POINTS

Use your thumb or your elbow to firmly massage the area shown. These lymphatics not only improve conditions of the intestinal tract but are also extremely useful for low back pain.

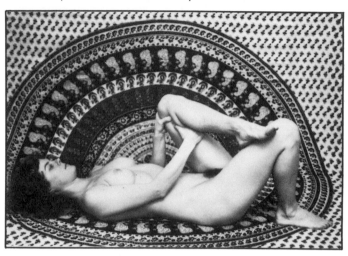

SMALL INTESTINE
Neuro-lymphatic Massage Points

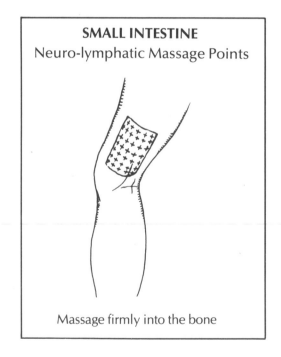

Massage firmly into the bone

CONSTIPATION
DIARRHEA LYMPHATICS

Use your knuckles to massage the outside of your thighs. Rub from the knee up to the hip to cure constipation and from the hip down to the knee to cure diarrhea. If your bowel movements are normal, rub up and down to encourage the continuation of normal bowel movements. Reverse recommendation if condition does not improve.

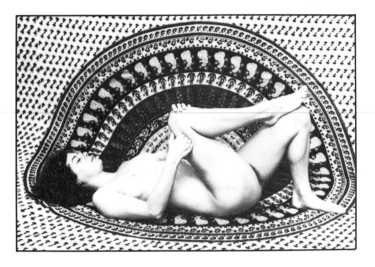

LIVER/SPLEEN/KIDNEY
SHINBONE PRESSURE POINT

Use your thumb to apply firm pressure for 3-5 seconds to the indicated point. All the functions of the above organs, as well as infections, respond to this pressure points.

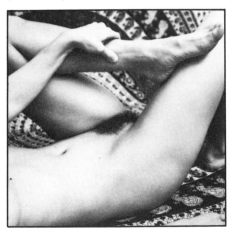

LEG TWIST

Use both hands and twist from below the ankle to the top of the thigh. This technique feels good, releases tension and helps to force stagnant blood and lymph out of the legs back to the heart.

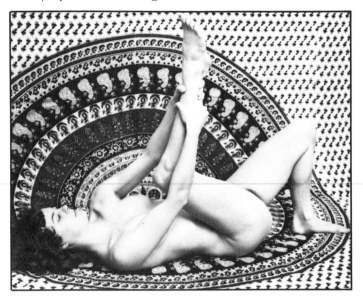

Do the other foot and leg before proceeding to the torso.

TORSO

ABDOMINAL MASSAGE

Begin a circular, sweeping massaging motion on the lower right side of the abdomen. Continue the motion up and across and then down to the lower left side of the abdomen. It is important to massage from right to left because the feces move in this direction. Repeat the circular massaging six times. Next, apply a firm penetrating pressure with four fingers into the abdomen. Begin at the lower right side and apply firm pressure every two inches. Always press in the direction of the fecal movement. When you reach the lower left side of the abdomen, vibrate and hold the last insertion for 10 seconds. This technique encourages healthy bowel movements.

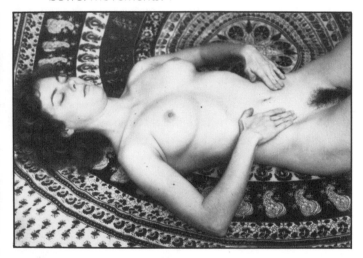

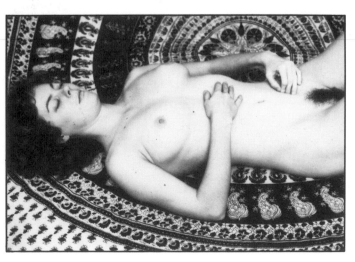

WAIST MASSAGE

This technique helps to trim the waistline and stimulates liver and gall bladder functions. With thumbs forward and fingers back, squeeze and twist the flesh while massaging. Alternate left and right.

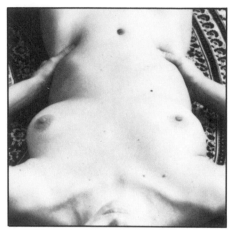

FOUR-FINGER RIB MASSAGE

Begin at the xiphoid process. Massage into the bottom edge of the rib cage from the xiphoid process to the waist and the lower back. Repeat, but this time gently massage under the rib cage to reach some of the internal organs. The functions of the liver, gall bladder, stomach, pancreas and small intestine can be improved by frequent utilization of this technique.

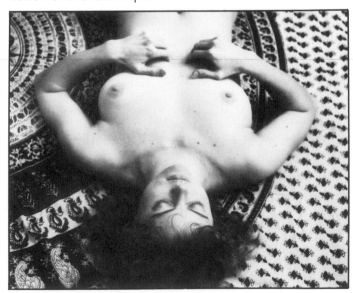

INTERCOSTAL RIB TRACING

Use four fingers and begin in the area of the lower back. Place each finger between two ribs, then press into the intercostal spaces and pull your fingers along, in these spaces, until you reach the sternum. Repeat two or three times, then proceed to trace the upper ribs. Do one side at a time. This technique flushes the lymphatic system and stimulates the intercostal muscles and nerves.

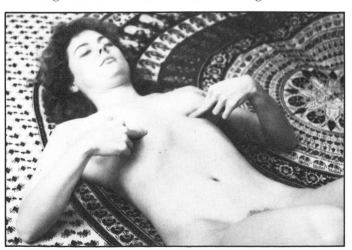

STOMACH/LIVER/ GALL BLADDER LYMPHATICS

Massage for 20-30 seconds, the intercostal spaces between the fifth and sixth ribs. These are located under the breasts or pectoralis muscles, on both the left and right sides of the torso. This improves digestion and disturbances of the digestive tract.

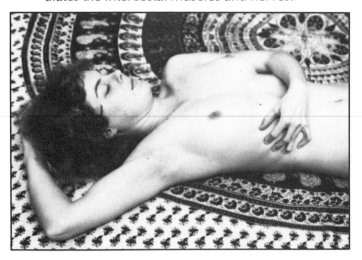

BREAST MASSAGE

Massage in small circular motions and feel for lumps as you do so. Cover both breasts thoroughly.

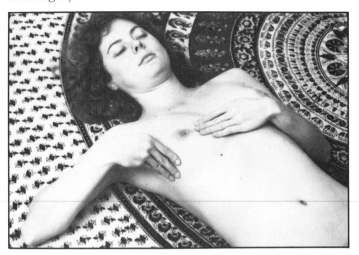

PECTORALIS MASSAGE

Massage for 5-10 seconds the origins and insertions of the pectoralis major clavicular and sternal muscles. This technique not only strengthens and firms the chest muscles but also helps to improve digestion.

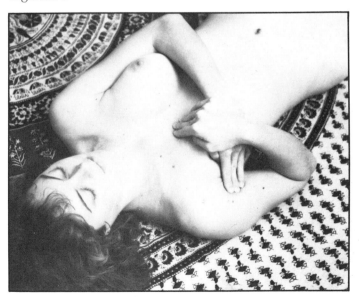

LUNG LYMPHATIC DRAINAGE TECHNIQUE

Massage the intercostal spaces between the third and fourth, then fourth and fifth ribs on both sides of the sternum. These points, which are located directly between the breasts or pectoralis muscles, should be done for 10-15 seconds.

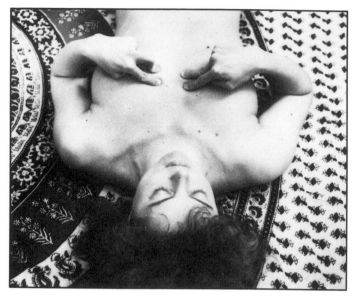

THYROID FUNCTION & HEART

Use your middle fingers to massage between the second and third ribs in the intercostal spaces next to the sternum. These lymphatic massage points help to regulate and normalize heart and thyroid functions.

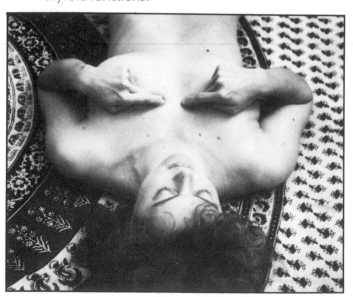

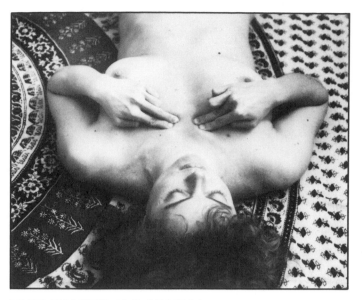

KIDNEY STIMULATION

Massage for 20-30 seconds the first ribs, which are located under the clavicle protuberances, in order to flush the neuro-lymphatic drainage system for the kidneys. Also, drink six to eight glasses of water daily to keep your kidneys functioning properly. Drink before meals or one-and-a-half to two hours after meals. Do not drink while eating as water dilutes your digestive juices.

BRAIN STIMULATION

Use your finger tips to massage thoroughly from the hollow found below the clavicles to the arm pits. Slow learners and people who experience brain fatigue find relief after two or three minutes of massaging these areas. For study purposes it necessary to repeat this technique every few hours, or more often in order to keep the circuits to the brain open and functioning.

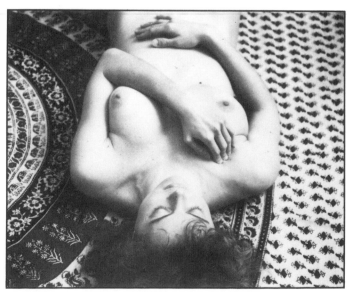

HANDS & ARMS

Massage one hand and arm before proceeding to the other.

FINGERTIP PINCH & TWIST

Grasp the base of each nail between your thumb and index finger. Firmly pinch and twist each finger for 7-10 seconds to stimulate the flow of energy along the meridians that terminate or begin at the nails of the hand.

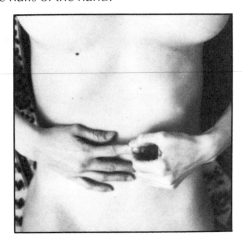

FINGER & THUMB MASSAGE

Massage your digits thoroughly from the tip to the palm. This technique forces stagnant blood back to the heart.

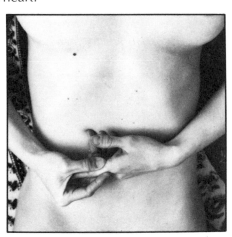

FOUR-FINGER MASSAGE

Position your fingers on the palm immediately below the fingers. Ten circular massaging motions over the bony protuberances in a clockwise direction will stimulate your eyes, ears, sinuses, teeth and brain. Your fingers must be relaxed when executing this technique.

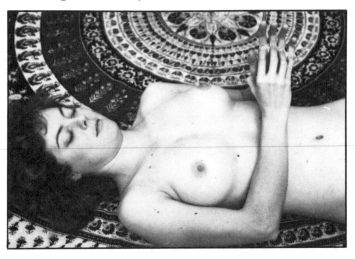

FOUR-FINGER METACARPAL SLIDE

Position your fingers in the grooves directly below the knuckles on the top of your hand. Slide your fingers across the top of your hand and over the wrist. Try to follow the grooves formed by the metacarpal bones. Three upward motions are sufficient to relax the hand and wrist.

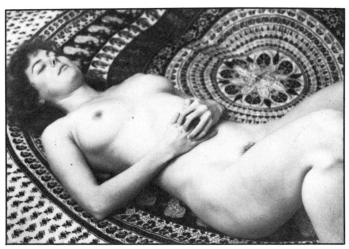

129

FOREARM ACUPUNCTURE PRESSURE POINTS

Use your thumb to press and hold each of the indicated points for 3-5 seconds. Repeat applications three times if you have a condition associated with these points.

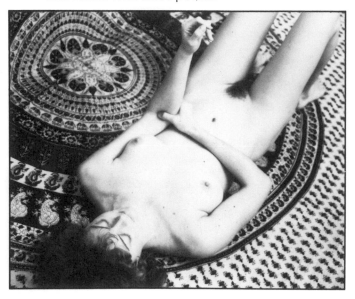

FOREARM PRESSURE POINTS

Circulation/Sexual & Reproductive organs

Heart

L5

H3

Lung

C/S3

L6

C/S4

C/S5

C/S6

L7

H4

H5

L8

H6

L9

H7

C/S7

Apply firm pressure

UPPER ARM MASSAGE

Use your entire hand to massage the biceps and triceps. Massage toward the heart and deep into the muscles of the upper arm. Then grasp the deltoid muscles and massage.
Repeat these techniques on the other hand and arm before proceeding to the neck and shoulders.

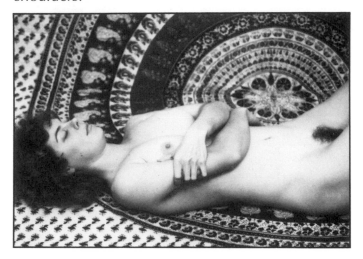

NECK & SHOULDERS

SHOULDER/UPPER TRAPEZIUS TENSION

Do this technique with your arms bent and alongside your chest. Massage the origin, insertion and belly of the upper trapezius muscle with your finger tips. Keep your shoulders relaxed as you massage.

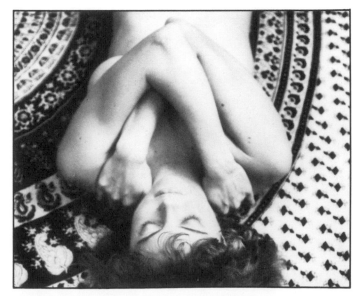

CERVICAL PRESSURE

Begin at the base of the neck. Apply firm pressure to both sides of the cervical vertebrae. Use your middle finger to apply the pressure. Brace it with the fingers on either side of it. Hold each application of pressure for 7-10 seconds.

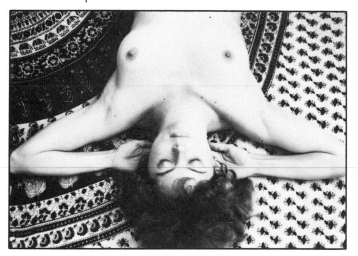

SHOULDER PRESSURE POINTS

Brace your middle finger as above. Beginning at the edge of the shoulder, work your way, with the middle finger, toward the neck and hold each application of pressure for 10 seconds. This technique relieves neck and shoulder tension. Keep your shoulders relaxed as you work.

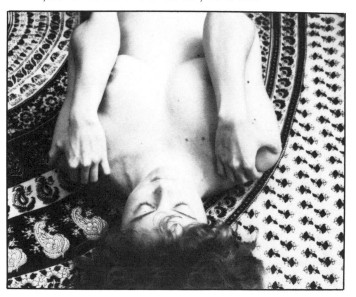

BASE OF THE SKULL PRESSURE POINTS

Use three fingers to apply firm penetrating pressure into the base of the skull. Hold each application of pressure for 10 seconds. Neck and shoulder tension as well as gall bladder conditions will benefit from the regular use of these points.

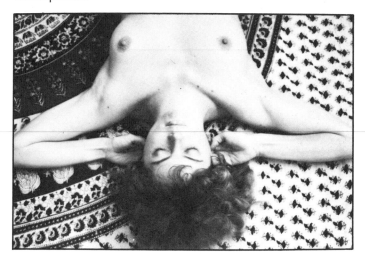

STERNOCLEIDOMASTOID MUSCLES OF THE NECK

Don't let the word throw you. The technique is simple. Use four fingers to massage the large muscle on each side of the neck. Using small circular motions, massage from under the ears to the clavicle protuberances. Do not apply too much pressure as this muscle is usually tender.

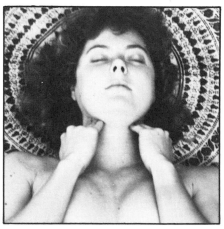

THYROID STIMULATION

Press gently alongside and slightly under the Adam's apple with three fingers for 7-10 seconds. Repeat both sides twice. The thyroid gland produces hormones that keep you looking young.

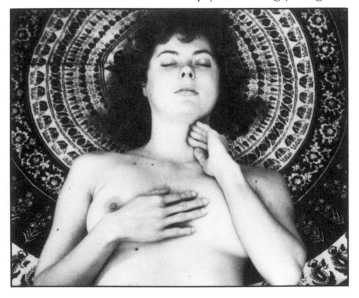

HEAD

SCALP MASSAGE

Using your finger tips or your fingernails, thoroughly massage the scalp. This technique encourages hair growth and improves scalp conditions.

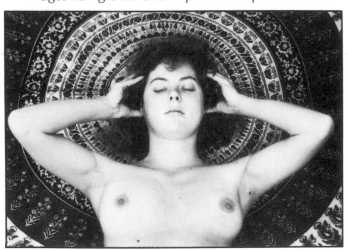

SINUS PRESSURE POINTS

Apply firm pressure with your middle finger as you move from the widow's peak to the top of the back of your head. Hold each application for 3-5 seconds.

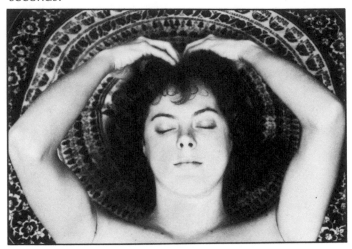

GALL BLADDER PRESSURE POINTS

Apply firm pressure to the Gall Bladder Meridian where it travels around the ear. Hold each pressure application for 3-5 seconds. This technique will benefit the gall bladder and your hearing.

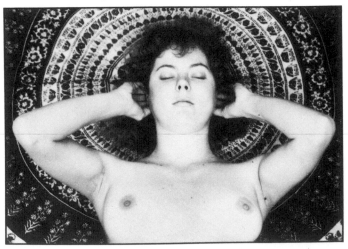

FACE

Use a little cream for the first three techniques.

FOREHEAD STROKE

Slide four fingers from your eyebrows up into the hairline. Repeat two or three times to relax the brow.

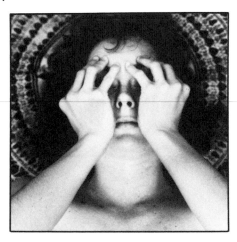

CHEEK MASSAGE

Slide four fingers from the chin up and out to the temples and into the hairline.

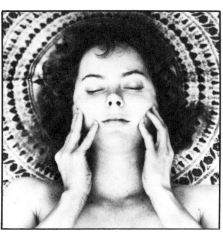

CHIN LINE TRIMMER

With your thumbs under your chin, alternately pull them toward the ears. Repeat two or three times if your chin line is good, ten times if your chin line sags.

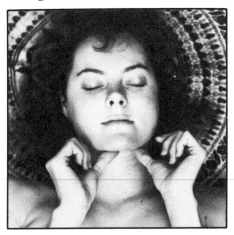

EYE SOCKET—UPPER RIDGE

Apply firm pressure for 3-5 seconds along the entire upper ridge of the eye socket. This technique improves eyesight, relieves eyestrain and benefits sinus conditions.

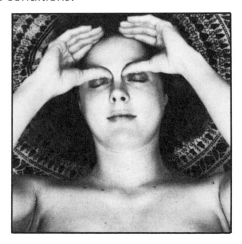

EYE SOCKETS—LOWER RIDGE

Use your index fingers to apply a firm pressure for 3-5 seconds to the entire lower ridge of the eye sockets. This technique yields the same benefits as the upper-ridge technique and also improves digestion.

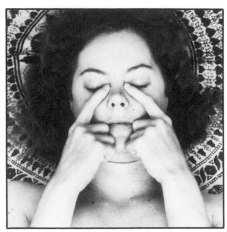

SINUS & LARGE INTESTINE POINTS

Apply a very firm thumb pressure for 3-5 seconds to the entire base of the cheekbones. Sinus as well as intestinal disturbances respond to frequent use of these points.

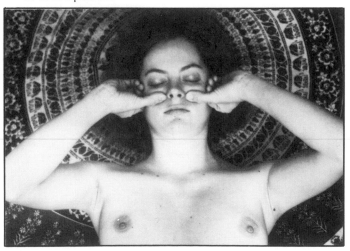

GUM MASSAGE

Use your fingers to massage first the upper and then the lower gums. This technique benefits your gums and the nerves of your teeth. If your gums bleed when you brush your teeth, massage your gums frequently and be sure to obtain additional vitamin C from fresh fruits and natural ascorbic acid supplements. Do not stretch or pull the skin. Lift your fingers off the skin before proceeding to the next area to be massaged.

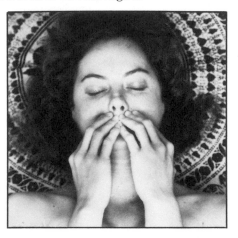

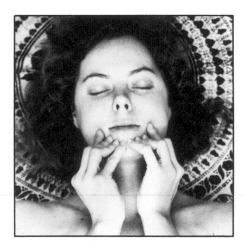

JAW TENSION

Use your thumbs or middle fingers to massage firmly the joints where the mandible meets the skull. Tension accumulates in this joint, but massage does much to relieve it.

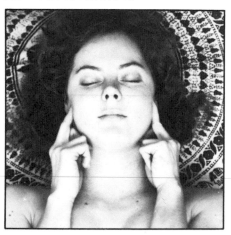

EYE MASK

Position your fingers lightly over your closed eyes for approximately 10 seconds. Do not press into your eyes. Simply rest your fingers lightly on them and allow the heat from your fingers to help relieve eye fatigue. Rub your hands together vigorously to warm your fingers prior to positioning them over your eyes.

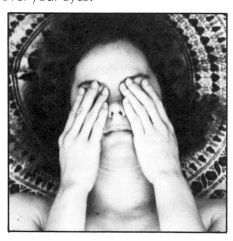

EARS

EAR MASSAGE

There are approximately fifty acupuncture points on each ear. Auricular therapy thus affects the whole body. By massaging, pulling and lightly pinching the ears, you are stimulating the entire body. Auricular therapy traditionally utilizes gold needles to strengthen, silver needles to sedate and stainless steel needles to balance the body's energies. Ear massage serves the body positively by improving its circulation and energy flow. Massaging the ears also feels wonderful. It may end up being one of your favorite techniques. Begin with the ear lobes, then work your way up and into the ears. Get into all the crevices. Massage, pull and pinch the entire ear. Gently and briefly insert your fingers into the orifice. Hold them there for a few seconds, then vibrate them lightly to stimulate the inner ear.

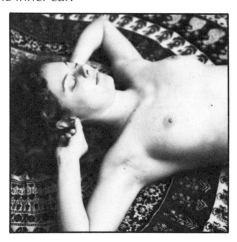

BACK

UPPER THORACIC VERTEBRAE

Use your middle fingers , braced by the fingers on either side of them to apply penetrating pressure to the side of and between the upper thoracic vertebrae. Massage the area where you applied pressure before moving on to the next pair of vertebrae.

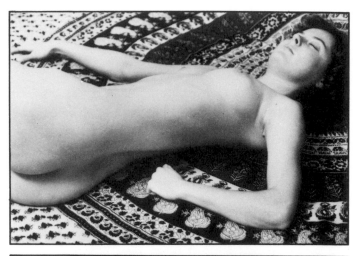

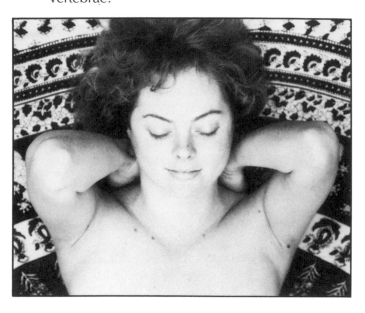

MIDDLE THORACIC VERTEBRAE

Do one side of the spine at a time. Lie on your back with your hip and leg to one side. Form a fist with your hand on the side of your raised hip. Position the most prominent knuckle alongside and between the highest pair of vertebrae you can reach. When the knuckle has been positioned, allow your back to rest on the knuckle. Apply firm pressure for 3-5 seconds, then massage the area with your knuckle. Return to the twisted position and locate the pair of vertebrae just below the one you have just worked. Repeat the technique. Continue in this manner until you reach the eleventh and twelfth thoracic vertebrae.

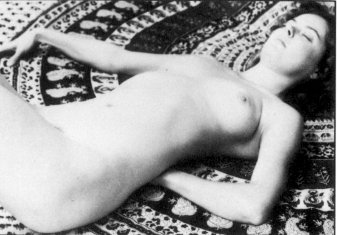

LUMBAR VERTEBRAE

Insert your hands, palms up and with your fingers bent, under your lower back. Use your middle fingers, braced with the fingers on either side of it, to apply firm pressure and then massage along the spine and between the vertebrae.

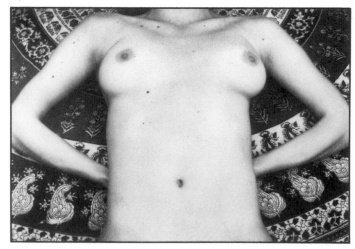

3) A MASSAGE PROGRAM FOR CHILDREN

It's natural for infants to touch and be touched. If a child is deprived of touch during early infancy, or at any other time in its development, physical as well as psychological disturbances are the result. The first twelve months of human life are critical. Adequate physical contact during the first year is of utmost importance for high levels of intelligence, for the proper functioning of internal organs and for emotional maturity. Give your child the opportunity to develop to her/his fullest potential. Begin massaging your child prenatally and continue through the various stages of develoment, including puberty and adolescence.

Massaging your child prior to birth may seem a little farfetched at first. When you think about it carefully, however, you'll see that it makes sense because touch and massage enhance the psychic union between the mother and her unborn child. Thus, the bond between them will be strengthened, as will their emotional health and stability.

The following photographs illustrate easily mastered techniques of massaging your child through the abdominal wall. A diagram also indicates what pressure/holding points are useful for encouraging a normal and healthy pregnancy, an easy delivery and ultimately, a vibrant baby.

CIRCULATION/SEX
Neuro-vascular Holding Points

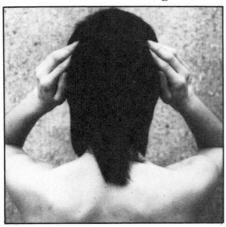

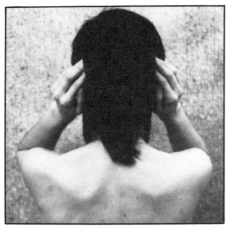

Hold lightly & feel for a pulse

CIRCULATION/SEX ACUPUNCTURE PRESSURE POINTS FOR A HEALTHY BABY

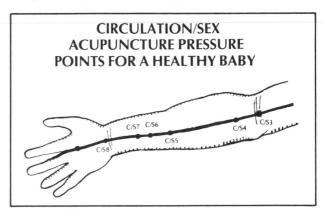

CLOCKWISE FULL HAND CIRCULAR MASSAGE
Lightly, slowly and sensitively glide your hands in a clockwise movement over the abdomen.

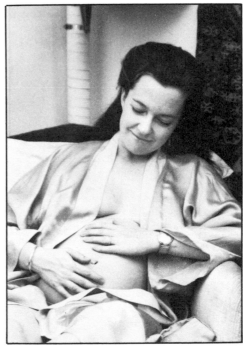

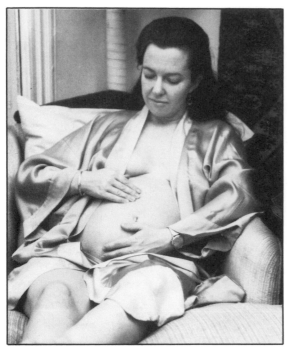

CIRCULAR KNEADING OF ABDOMEN
Stabilize abdomen with one hand and *gently*
knead, with slow, small, slightly penetrating circular
movements. Switch hands and repeat technique
on the other side of abdomen.

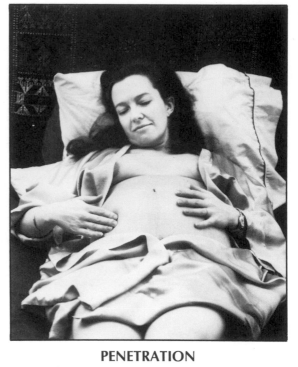

PENETRATION
Use four fingers as one; *slowly* and *gently*
penetrate the abdominal wall in numerous places
while the other hand is a stabilizer.

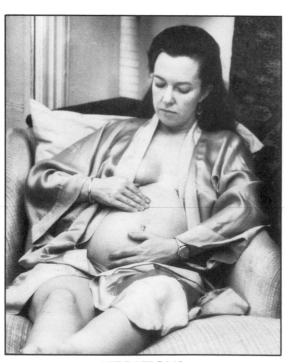

VIBRATIONS
Gently vibrate the abdominal wall in many
locations by using four fingers as one.

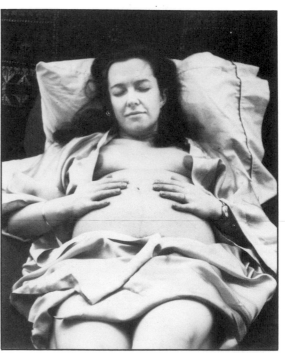

SENSATIONS
Lay your full hands over the abdomen, focus your
attention and communicate with your baby.
Listen, feel and observe.

Massaging after birth will continue to develop and strengthen the bond between parents and child. It is especially useful to parents who work outside the home, for long daily absences almost inevitably lead to some estrangement of the parents from the child. What better way is there to keep in touch than to massage your child briefly before bed?

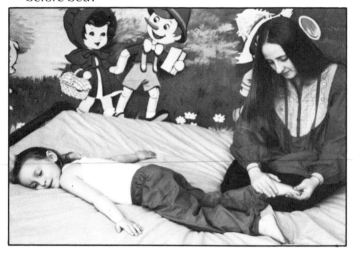

Many children are eager to learn massage and are quite capable of giving one. Encourage your child to massage you on occasion. As young children can easily be overwhelmed by the immensity of an adult body, suggest that your child massage only one part of your body, such as your face, or perhaps one hand or foot. Massage is a highly effective method of strengthening and maintaining the love, trust and compassion between you and your child.

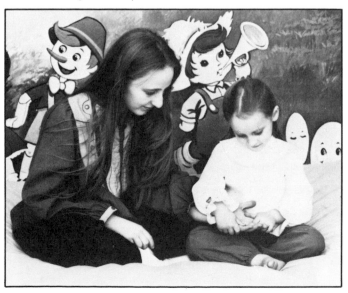

Massage for children can be approached in several different ways. You can set aside one day a week for a Complete 60-Minute Body Massage, you can utilize your favorite techniques frequently throughout the week, you can use specific techniques as they are required, or, you can combine all of the above approaches.

The Complete 60-Minute Body Massage can be readily adapted to a massage routine that is very pleasurable and healthful to children of all ages. The most important thing to remember when massaging a child is that children require less pressure than adults to reap the same benefits from massage. As children are also generally more open to massage than most adults, their young bodies will respond optimally to light or medium pressure. NEVER apply firm pressure. A young child will not understand why you are hurting her or him, and consequently will develop a dislike for massage. If necessary, when you want to relieve a toothache, for example, you can explain to an older child that although a technique may hurt a little, the pain will help the ache to go away. Good pain hurts a little but helps a lot!

Children who are still small enough to rest on your extended legs during a massage should receive the following <u>reordered</u>, altered and somewhat abbreviated version of the Complete 60-Minute Body Massage. Once a child grows too tall or weighs too much to lie comfortably on your legs, you can implement the Complete 60-Minute Body Massage; but rather than using the heel or whole of your hand, use only two or three fingers or a long thumb.

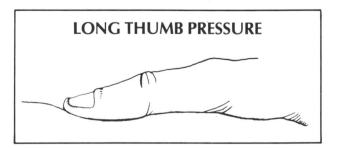

LONG THUMB PRESSURE

You as the doer, can either sit on an armless, straight-back chair with your legs raised and extended on another chair, or else on a bed or on the floor with your legs stretched out. As the ability to move your arms freely is important, place several pillows behind your back. This provides the doer support for the back, which is important as it prevents fatigue and low back pain.

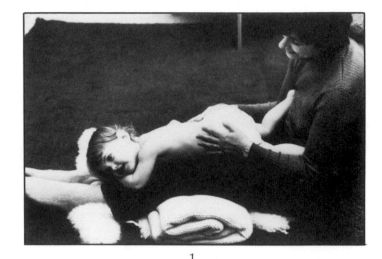

1

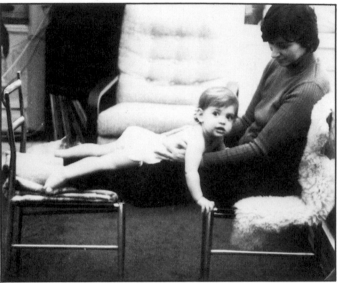

The child can be placed in four possible positions. The first is prone (face down) and lying parallel to and on the doer's legs. Be sure either to turn the child's head comfortably to the side or to allow space between and below your legs so the child can breathe easily. Sitting in a chair with your legs raised on another chair assures the child necessary air, but if you feel more comfortable on the floor or on a bed, raise your legs slightly at the thigh and ankle with pillows in order to create the needed air space. The second position is supine (face up) and lying parallel to and on the doer's legs with the child's head towards the doer's feet. In the third position, the child also lies supine and parallel to the doer's legs, but this time the child's head is near the doer's abdomen. Finally, in the fourth position, the child lies prone and perpendicular across the doer's thighs. If you simply cannot work in any of these positions, improvise until you find one that suits both you and your child. Always be concerned, however, with your comfort and the child's ability to breathe.

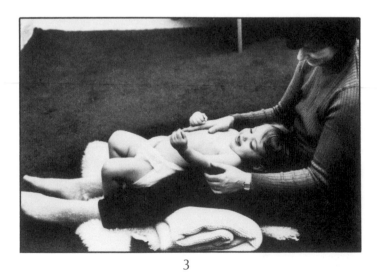

2

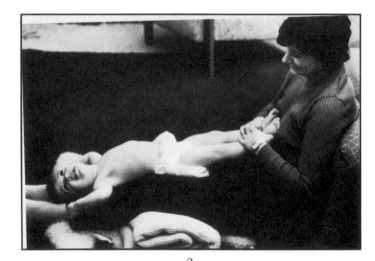

3

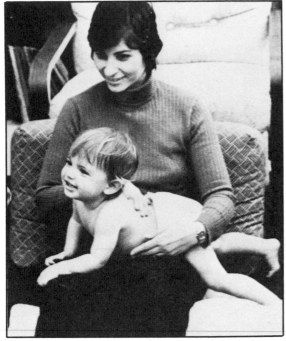

4

Section 6 of this chapter provides photographs of the techniques that are useful for common childhood conditions and complaints. Once again, remember that the techniques are always to be performed with light or medium pressure. These pressure points can be used as a preventive measure or as an adjunct to your doctor's suggestions for treatment of the condition.

A MASSAGE PROGRAM FOR CHILDREN WHO ARE STILL SMALL ENOUGH TO LIE ON YOUR EXTENDED LEGS

TECHNIQUE #1: The First Touch consists of picking up, kissing, hugging and then positioning the child on your legs in the supine position with the child's head away from your abdomen.
Then proceed to Technique #31 of the Complete 60-Minute Body Massage.

Unfortunately, in an attempt to keep the price of this book within range of most people's budgets, I cannot detail each technique as I did in the Complete 60-Minute Body Massage. The following pages, however, have been dotted to indicate a cutting line so that you can, if you choose to, remove them and have them readily accessible when using the Complete 60-Minute Body Massage as your guide.

When referring to the Complete 60-Minute Body Massage while massaging your child, concern yourself primarily with the *Technique* sections. Be certain to use only light pressure and gentle kneading on children. *Purpose* may or may not concern you, for you may be using the techniques simply to make the child feel good. As for *Repetition*, let your instincts dictate how often you repeat a technique. The massage program for small children should be flexible with respect to time. Less than an hour or more than an hour is fine. Finally, *Positioning* is of no importance because your position and that of the child are unique to this massage program for small children.

Do what comes naturally. Touch and massage your child to better physical, intellectual and emotional health. It's never too late to begin. Children of all ages will respond favorably to the introduction of massage into their daily routine.

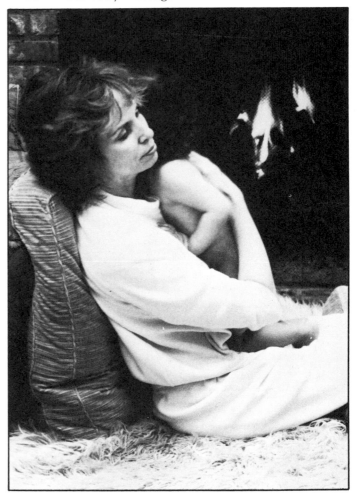

TECHNIQUES #31–39: No changes, but don't forget to repeat Technique #32–37 on the other foot before proceeding to the next technique.

TECHNIQUE #40: Omit.

TECHNIQUES #41–49: No changes, except in Technique #46 use three fingers.

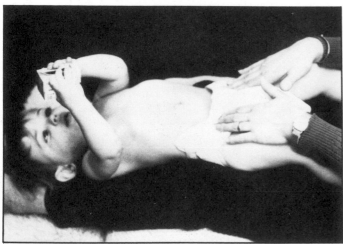

46) PUBIC LYMPH DRAINAGE

TECHNIQUE #50: Omit.

TECHNIQUES #51–54: Use index finger.

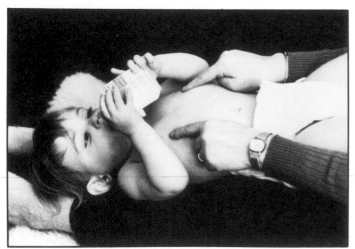

51) LIVER & STOMACH LYMPHATIC DRAINAGE

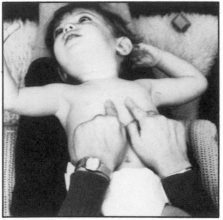

52) LUNG LYMPHATIC DRAINAGE

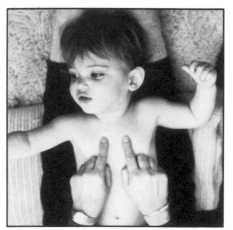

53) HEART & THYROID LYMPHATIC POINTS

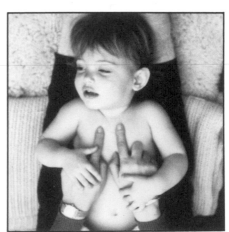

54) KIDNEY LYMPHATIC DRAINAGE

TECHNIQUE #55: Omit.

TECHNIQUES #56–63: No changes, but in Technique #56 use three fingers and in #63 use the long thumb. Don't forget to repeat Techniques #56–63 on the other arm.

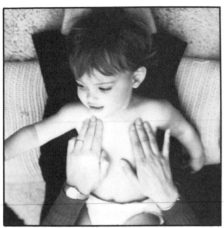

56) SHOULDER KNEADING

TECHNIQUES #64–66: Omit.

TECHNIQUES #67–73: The only change is that of position. Reposition the child supine (face up), with the child's head near your abdomen.

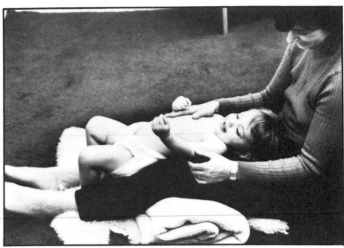

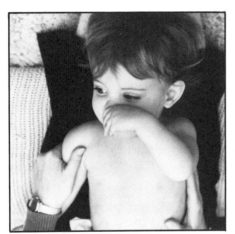

63) UPPER ARM LUNG
MERIDIAN PRESSURE

TECHNIQUE #74: Omit.

TECHNIQUES #75–81: No changes.

TECHNIQUES #82–85: Omit.

TECHNIQUES #86–93: No changes.

TECHNIQUES #94–103: No changes, but in Technique #103 use two fingers.

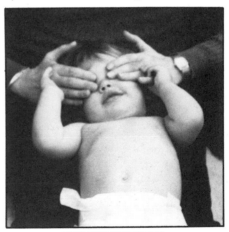

103) EYE PRESSURE

TECHNIQUES #1–2: Omit.

TECHNIQUE #3: Use the index and middle fingers.

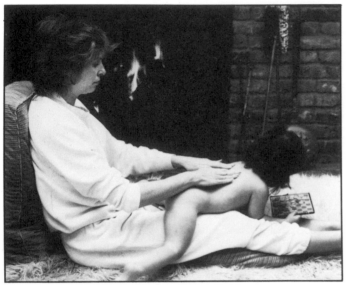

3) SPINE TRACING

Now turn the child over in a prone position for the following techniques. Lay the child perpendicularly across your thighs.

TECHNIQUE #4: Use four fingertips of both hands.

4) ROCKING THE BACK

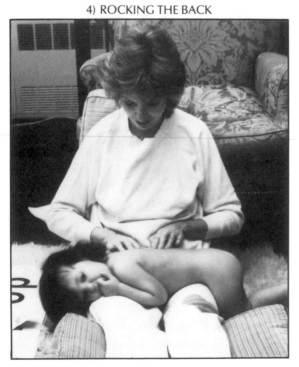

TECHNIQUE #5: Omit.

TECHNIQUES #6–10: Change positioning so that the child is still lying prone (face down), but with the head closer to your knees or ankles. Don't forget to allow for breathing space.

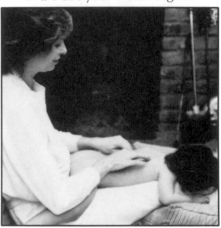

In #6 use your index fingers.

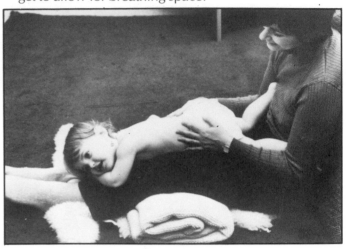

6) VERTEBRAE TECHNIQUE

In #10 use three fingertips together.

10) KNEADING OF THE BUTTOCK

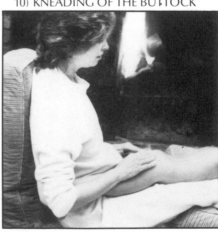

TECHNIQUES #11–14: No change, except in #11 and #13 use the full thumb.

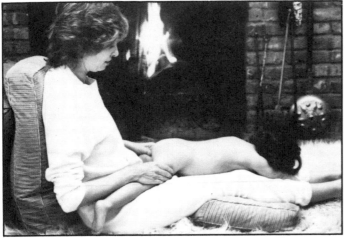

11) THIGH BLADDER MERIDIAN PRESSURE

#26–27 require no change.
#28 should be executed with two or three fingers.

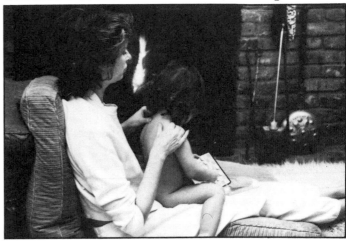

28) SHOULDER KNEADING

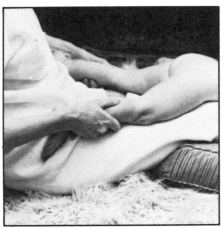

13) LOWER BACK OF THE LEG
BLADDER MERIDIAN PRESSURE

TECHNIQUES #15–21: No changes.

TECHNIQUES #22–30: #22–24 no change.
#25 should be executed with the index fingers.

25) UPPER THORACIC VERTEBRAE TECHNIQUE

#30 implements movements upward from the coccyx to the head.

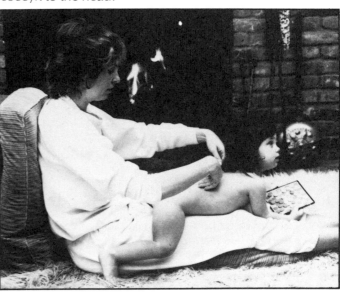

30) FEATHERING THE SPINE

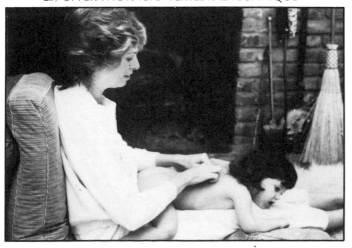

4) HOW TO GIVE A NEURO-VASCULAR MASSAGE

Neuro-vascular holding points or receptors, used regularly, are excellent health enhancers. They improve the circulation, especially that of the capillaries, and as you know, anything that improves the circulation improves overall physical and emotional well-being. Impaired circulation, which may be the result of a sedentary life style or poor eating habits or possibly a hereditary predisposition for circulatory disorders, will, over a period of years, greatly reduce the body's ability to function optimally. The body's many organs and systems require a constant supply of nutrients and oxygen in order to repair themselves and to maintain a healthy internal equilibrium.

Improved capillary circulation will also greatly benefit the body's largest organ, the skin. Acne, pallor (extreme or unnatural paleness), dry or oily skin and lifeless hair are but some of the conditions that improve through the regular use of neuro-vascular holding points. Such important body functions as digestion, elimination and respiration also benefit from neuro-vascular massage. Furthermore, improved circulation facilitates the endocrine glands' production of hormones, which regulate the growth, reproduction and nutrient utilization of the body's cells. This, in turn, insures or encourages adequate or optimal cellular activity, normal growth patterns in the formative years and healthy reproductive organs that will permit the continuation and forward the development of a healthy and superior species.

Neuro-vascular holding points are capable of affecting the organs in another important way too.

Our bodies are constantly confronted with toxins, not only those produced within the body, but also those ingested through the digestive tract and inhaled through the respiratory system. Toxins must be continually removed in order for the body to maintain its delicate balance known as homeostasis. An accumulation of toxic wastes within the system impairs bodily functions and can, when excessive, result in death. Improved circulation effects the speedy elimination of backed-up toxic materials and thus allows the body to resume its activities. Lactic acid, a waste that accumulates in the muscles after physical activity, illness or extended periods of inactivity due to a sedentary life style, must also be released. Physical exercise is, of course, the best way to release these toxins. When, however, exercise is not possible or when a supplement to exercise is required, the neuro-vascular holding points are extremely useful and can be included in a full body massage program.

Execution of the neuro-vascular massage is extremely easy, and whether done by yourself or someone else, it is gratifying. If you do the points yourself, there are two possible positions you can assume. One possibility is a reclining position. Lie in bed or on the floor with your knees propped up by pillows or bolster cushions, and support your arms with additional pillows. The second possibility is a crouched position, which is also assumed on a bed or on the floor. Place a folded towel or small compact pillow between your forehead and the floor or bed. Some people find this position easier because the arms are completely relaxed and supported. If you find crouching forward uncomfortable, use the reclining position.

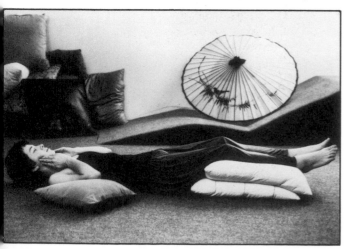

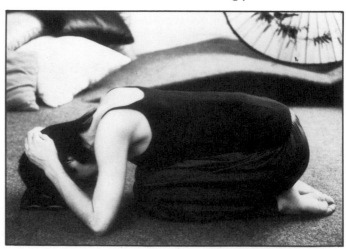

If someone is doing the points for you, refer to the photographs for the most comfortable position. If you are doing the points yourself, be sure your arms are sufficiently propped or supported to prevent the development of muscular fatigue, which will spoil the relaxing and beneficial effects of the neuro-vascular massage.

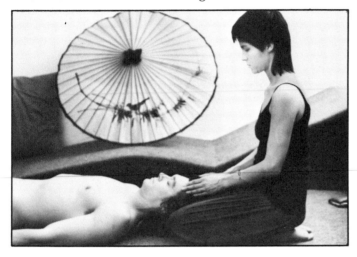

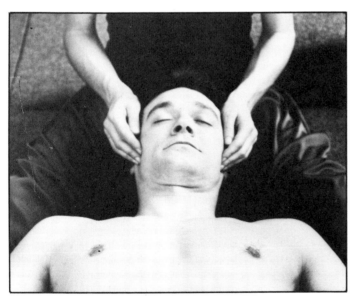

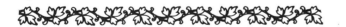

IMPORTANT CONSIDERATIONS FOR THE NEURO-VASCULAR MASSAGE

- Remove contact lenses.

- Breathe slowly and regularly.

- Make contact with the points by using a light pressure.

- While holding the points, try to keep calm and perfectly still because the slightest movement or turn of the head sends vibrations down your arm which are felt by the receiver.

- Withdraw from the points slowly so as not to jar the receiver.

- If you notice the receiver's eyes batting, it is a sign that the receiver is thinking. Quietly suggest that the receiver try not to think.

- Use the pads of your fingers, not your fingertips.

CORRECT

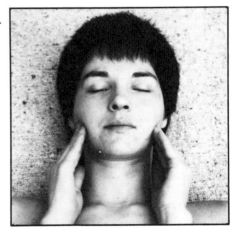

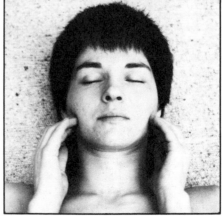

INCORRECT

What to do is extremely simple. Study the following photographs to locate the neuro-vascular holdings points. Feel for a very delicate subcutaneous pulse, i.e. a faint beat under the skin. Hold the pulse for 20-30 seconds and then move on to the next pair of points. Not all the points are found in pairs. Follow the numerical sequence indicated in the photographs. After five or six sessions with the points, you will probably remember their location and sequence so that you will no longer need the book as a guide. The pulses should be held gently and withdrawal must be executed slowly.

Don't be surprised if you fall asleep during this process. You may also notice that you twitch, snore, make nonsensical sounds or release short spurts of words that may or may not make sense. These are all good signs, for they indicate that you are letting go and releasing stored tension.

If someone is doing your points for you, you are more likely to fall asleep because you won't have to concern yourself with maintaining contact with the points. Encourage yourself to relax and let go. Try to free your mind from thought. If you find that impossible, allow thoughts to flow through your mind in a stream of consciousness. Do not focus on any of the thoughts or images, but simply allow them to pass through your mind's eye. Many people have reported achieving a transcendental state of being during neuro-vascular massage. Some people say they feel as if they are floating in and out of consciousness, while others say they have the sensation that they are no longer lying on the mat but floating slightly above it. You may also feel waves of relaxation sweeping over your entire body or through its various parts. If you are really in touch with your body, you may even be able to feel a rush of energy to the organ that corresponds to the points being held. Whatever you feel, it will undoubtedly be a very relaxing and fulfilling experience that you will want to repeat frequently.

The entire process will consume only 10 minutes of your time, and the effects will be well worth your while. You will feel as if you have been off on a long vacation. Your mental alertness will be renewed, your emotional balance restored and your physical well-being refreshed.

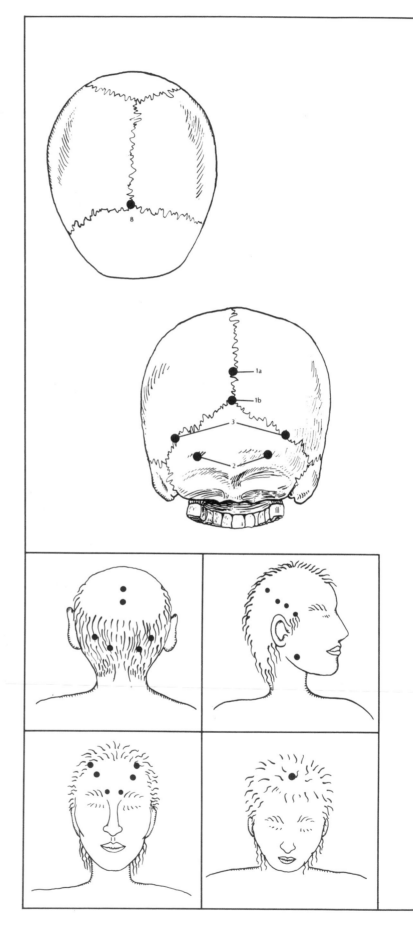

NEURO-VASCULAR HOLDING POINTS

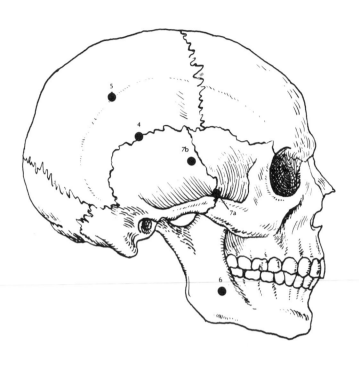
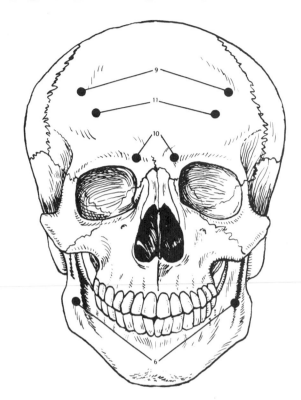

1a Posterior sagittal suture

1b Posterior fontanel

2 Occipital protuberance

3 Lambdoidal suture

4 Squamous suture

5 Parietal eminence

6 Ramus of the jaw

7a Temporal/Sphenoid juncture

7b Squamous portion of temporal bone

8 Anterior fontanel

9 Lateral frontal bone

10 Glabella

11 Frontal eminence

1a Infections, Fevers, Sore throat, Anemia, Tennis elbow

1b Large intestine (diarrhea, constipation, hem-morhoids, etc.), Adrenal Glands (ENERGY STABI-LIZATION), STRESS CONTROL, Fatigue, Blood sugar problems, Asthma, Allergies, Infection SHOCK from physical or emotional trauma

2 Kidneys, Restlessness, Skin conditions, Low back pain

3 Reproductive/Sexual organ conditions, Hormonal disturbances

4 Spleen, Allergies, Blood sugar problems

5 Small/Large intestine & Digestive disturbances, Kidneys, Reproductive/Sexual organ conditions

6 Stomach, Digestion, Sinus, Eyes, Nose

7a Kidney, Neck

7b Hyper/Hypothyroidism, NERVOUS SYSTEM, Spine

8 Gall Bladder, Liver, Heart & Lung conditons, BRAIN FATIGUE

9 Liver conditions, Headaches

10 Bladder functions & conditions

11 Stomach, Digestion, Bladder conditons, STRESS CONTROL

5) MASSAGE FOR COMMON
CHILDHOOD & ADULT COMPLAINTS

Below are some of the various points associated with many everyday complaints. Pain is an alarm system, the body's signal that some function is impaired or threatened. Always consult a holistically oriented physician as soon as you are able, for immediate attention can correct an imbalance before it becomes overwhelming. Use these points to ease any pain or release a blockage until you have the opportunity to consult your doctor, or use them as adjuncts to your doctor's recommendations. These points stimulate the body's natural healing mechanism and thus help to speed up your recovery.

See Neuro-lymphatic Massage Points Chart on page 46, Neuro-vascular Holding Points chart on pages 148 & 149, Meridian Acupuncture Reference Chart on pages 38 & 39 and Foot Reflexology Charts on page 67 & 79 for precise locations of the points utilized in this chapter.

HEADACHE

Each point indicated in the accompanying photographs relates to a particular type of headache. If you are uncertain of the origin of the headache or if the points you have chosen don't seem to be helping, simply do all the points. Trial and error will take care of your headache.

LIVER & GALL BLADDER
Neuro-lymphatic Massage Points

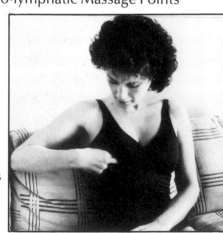

between the 5th & 6th ribs on the right side only

GALL BLADDER
Acupuncture Pressure points

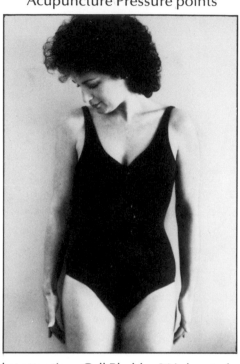

Stand at attention. Gall Bladder 31 is located where the fingertips touch the outside of the thigh.

STOMACH
Neuro-vascular Holding Points

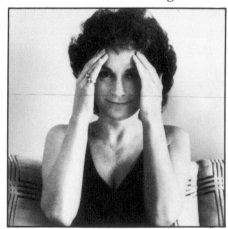

Hold the prominent bulges on your forehead (frontal eminence).

EYESTRAIN

Use your thumbs for the upper orbit and your fingers for the lower orbit of each eye. Apply pressure and hold for 3-5 seconds. Lymphatic massage points are located on the inside edge of the humerus bone. Use your thumb for these points.

UPPER ORBIT PRESSURE POINTS

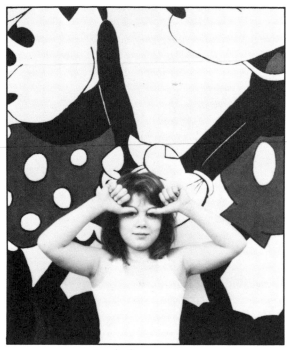

Apply firm pressure

KIDNEY
Neuro-lymphatic Massage Points

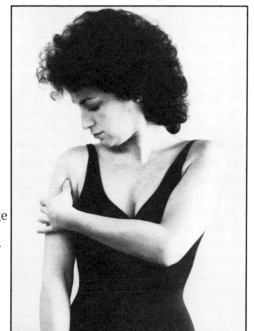

Massage both arms.

INDIGESTION

Indigestion can result from the malfunctioning of one or more of several digestive organs. Note the photographs for the exact location of each of the points. Apply pressure or massage the appropriate area(s) until you experience relief. Sometimes a period of as much as two to five minutes is necessary to relieve the discomfort. These points may also be stimulated prior to and during a meal in order to assist the deficient organ(s) and possibly to avoid indigestion.

STOMACH
Neuro-lymphatic Massage Points

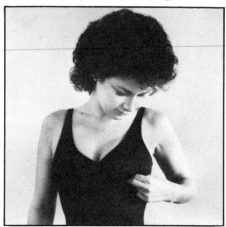

between the 5th & 6th ribs on the left side only

LIVER & GALL BLADDER
Neuro-lymphatic Massage Points

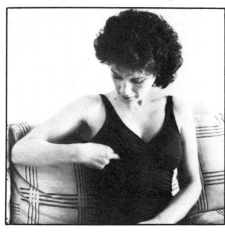

between the 5th & 6th ribs on the right side only

151

LOW BACK PAIN

The neuro-lymphatics for the lower back are located on the inside of the thigh. Use your elbow or your fingers to massage thoroughly and with a firm pressure the entire area depicted in the accompanying photograph. Usually one to three minutes are required to bring relief, although sometimes relief comes in thirty seconds.

SMALL INTESTINE
Neuro-lymphatic Massage Points

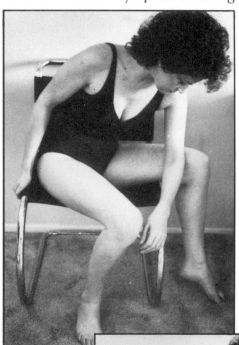

Massage firmly the lower half of the inside of the thigh.

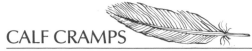

CALF CRAMPS

When you experience cramps or spasms in your calf muscle, you want to relax or sedate the mechanisms within the belly of the muscle. Feathering from the belly of the muscle toward the origin and insertion will sedate the muscle sufficiently to stop the spasm. Feathering is a very light technique. Try to evoke the same sensations a feather would if it were drawn over your calf muscle. It is not necessary to grab the muscle or to massage it deeply. Feathering stops the spasm sooner and with less effort than deep massage.

FEATHERING

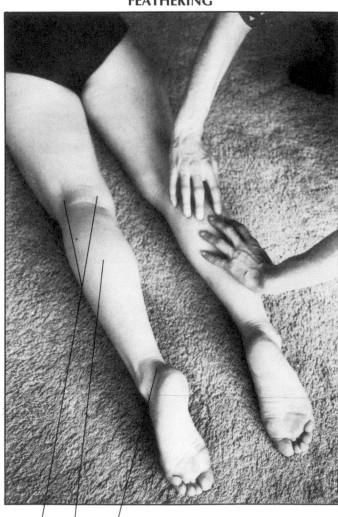

Origin   Belly   Insertion

TENNIS ELBOW

This common tennis injury is sometimes more complicated than you would expect. If the neuro-vascular holding points and the neuro-lymphatic massage points shown in the following photographs do not correct the conditions, you may well have a sacral fixation. Try bringing your knees up to your chest and rolling from side to side on the floor. If, after a reasonable time, no results are achieved, see a chiropractor.

SPLEEN
Neuro-lymphatic Massage Point

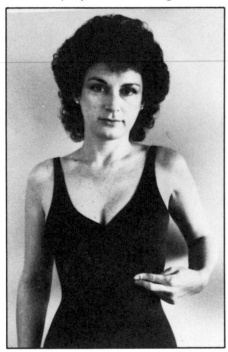

between the 7th & 8th ribs on the left side only

SPLEEN
Neuro-vascular Holding Point

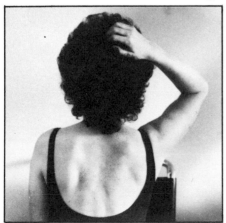

Locate this point 1½ inches above the posterior fontanel.

LOW ENERGY

Massage the two sets of points indicated in the photographs. One-and-a-half minutes for each set of points will usually be sufficient to clear a foggy mind and to supply you with more energy. These points are useful for long-distance driving, for studying, for sleepy attacks at concerts or for any occasion that would normally drive you to coffee. The points in the first set are located two-and-a-half inches above and one inch on either side of the navel. Massage deep into the abdomen, just below the rib cage. These points stimulate the functioning of your adrenal glands. Do not massage the adrenal points too close to bedtime because you may find yourself unable to sleep. The points of the second set are located on either side of the chest from the clavicle to the arm pit. Massage these neuro-lymphatics firmly, even though they may feel tender or a bit painful. The sensitivity will decrease as your alertness increases. These points correspond to the brain.

TRIPLE WARMER
Neuro-lymphatic Massage Points

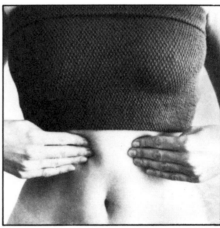

Locate these points under the rib cage.

CENTRAL
Neuro-lymphatic Massage Points

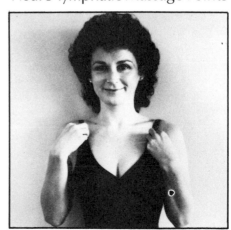

SORE THROAT

Below you will find three different approaches for deterring the progress or speeding the recovery of a sore throat. The neuro-lymphatic massage point for the throat is located on the left side of the chest between the seventh and eighth ribs. The point will be tender when you massage it, so you will know when you are in the correct location. The neuro-vascular holding point for a sore throat is located one-half inches above the Posterior fontanel, which was the baby soft spot on the back of the head. See Illustrations on pages 148 & 149 for the location of this point. Use the pads of your fingers to locate the point on your head. Be sure you feel a pulse under the scalp, and then hold this point for 1-3 minutes at a time as needed. The foot reflex point for a sore throat is located at the base of the big toe on the bottom of each foot. This point will also be tender to a firm touch. Be brave. Massage the base of the big toe with a very firm pressure. Try to endure the discomfort because the pain you may feel from the toe is going to be of a much shorter duration than that from the sore throat. These reflex points are particularly effective if used at the first sign of a sore throat. Use the points frequently, every fifteen minutes if necessary, and you may not even get a sore throat. If you begin to implement the points after the sore throat has settled in, you can achieve a speedier recovery, but usually cannot make it disappear.

Neuro-vascular Holding Point

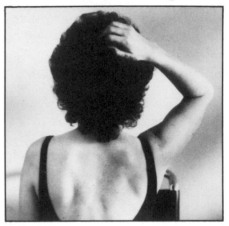

Located 1¹/₂ inches above the Posterior fontanel

FOOT REFLEXOLOGY

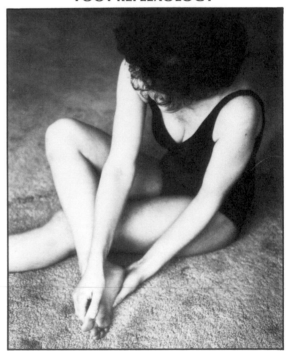

Massage firmly.

SPLEEN
Neuro-lymphatic Massage Point

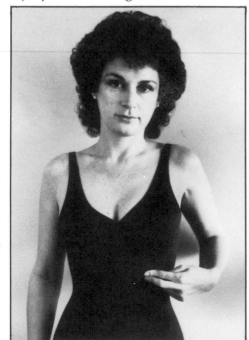

between the 7th & 8th ribs on the left side only

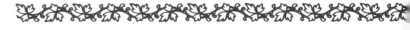

TOOTHACHE

Firmly massage and apply pressure to the inside edge of the humerus bone. If your toothache is on the right side of your mouth, massage your right arm; if it's on the left side, massage your left arm. You will undoubtedly find an extremely painful spot on the inside edge of your arm bone. That's the point. Work it hard. It will hurt, but the pain in your tooth will usually disappear in one or two minutes. The photograph shows a dark band of points. Try all of them. Usually one or two of these points will be more painful than the rest. These are the points on which to concentrate your pressure and massage. Be sure to consult your dentist. Remember, pain is the body's alarm system letting you know something is not right.

KIDNEY
Neuro-lymphatic Massage Points

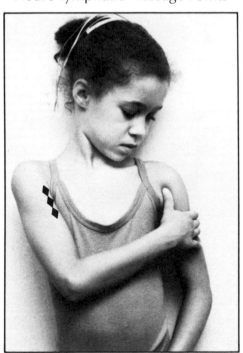

Massage firmly.

SMOKER'S LUNG

Massage the lymphatic points on either side of the sternum between the third and fourth as well as the fourth and fifth ribs, and/or apply firm pressure to each of the points indicated on the forearm for 7-10 seconds. Heavy smokers of cigarettes or marijuana should do these points four to six times a day.

LUNG
Neuro-lymphatic Massage Points

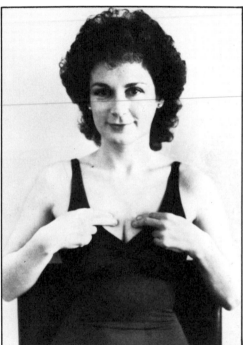

Massage near the sternum.

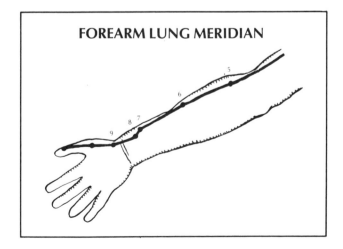

FOREARM LUNG MERIDIAN

DRINKER'S LIVER

Massage the intercostal space between the fifth and sixth ribs on the right side of the chest only. Use firm pressure and massage for 2-3 minutes four to six times a day. You may also hold the neuro-vascular point on the top of your head for 1-3 minutes four to six times a day. This technique helps to increase the flow of blood, nutrients and energy to your liver.

LIVER
Neuro-lymphatic Massage Points

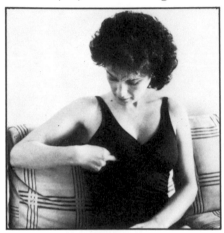

between the 5th & 6th ribs on the right side only

LIVER
Neuro-vascular Holding Point

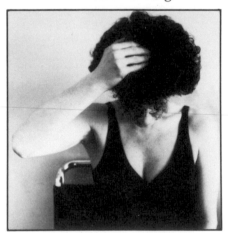

Locate this point on the Anterior fontanel
(baby's soft spot on top of the head)

CONSTIPATION/DIARRHEA

Thoroughly massage, with a firm pressure, the area indicated on the side of the thigh. Massage up to eliminate constipation and down to eliminate diarrhea. Massage when attempting to move your bowels, as well as once in the morning and once in the evening before going to sleep. Of course, plenty of bran, exercise and water are also factors important to proper functioning of the bowels.

LARGE INTESTINE
Neuro-lymphatic Massage Points

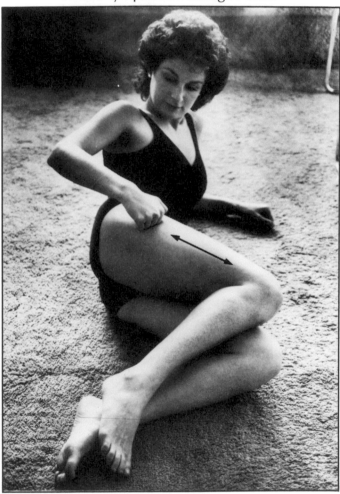

Massage both legs

SLEEPLESSNESS

Hold the neuro-vascular holding points located on the forehead. Feel for the pulse and hold the points for five minutes or longer. Usually within a few minutes you will begin to feel relaxed enough to fall asleep. You can also sedate your adrenal glands by holding the neuro-vascular holding point on the posterior fontanel. See page 149 for more information.

STOMACH
Neuro-vascular Holding Points

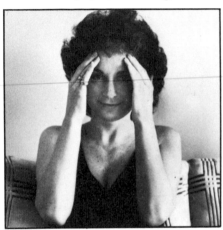

The frontal eminence points affect the emotional center of the brain

TRIPLE WARMER
Neuro-vascular Holding Point

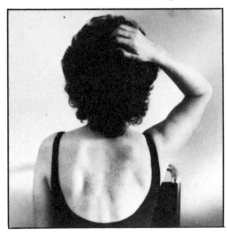

Locate this point on the posterior fontanel

SINUS CONDITIONS

Firmly massage the upper inner edge of the arm's humerus bone. Pressure applied to the orbits of the eyes also benefits sinus conditions. Firm pressure to the maxilla bones on either side of the nose is also very beneficial. Helpful too, are Large Intestine 20, and Lung 11. Hold each application of pressure for 7-10 seconds.

KIDNEY
Neuro-lymphatic Massage Points

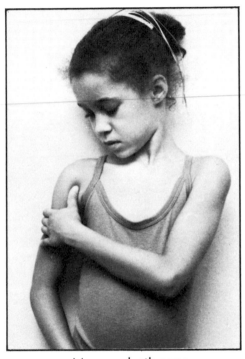

Massage both arms

LOWER ORBIT PRESSURE POINTS

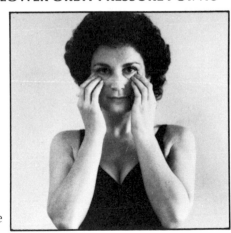

Apply firm pressure

LARGE INTESTINE
Acupuncture Pressure Points

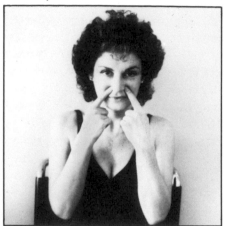

Apply firm pressure to Large intestine 20

LARGE INTESTINE & LUNG
Acupuncture Pressure Points

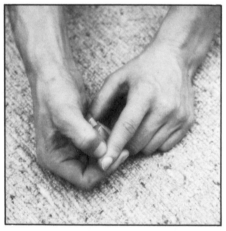

Apply firm
pressure to
Large intestine 1

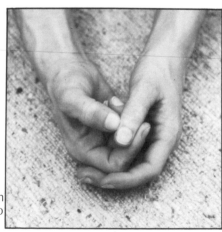

Apply firm
pressure to
Lung 11

SHOULDER & NECK TENSION

The following acupuncture points can be used with very firm thumb pressure for 7-10 seconds and repeated three times: Gall Bladder 20, Gall Bladder 21, Large Intestine 16 and Small Intestine 11. Of course, massaging the origin, belly and insertion of the upper trapezius muscle will also contribute to the release of shoulder and neck tension.

GALL BLADDER
Acupuncture Pressure Points

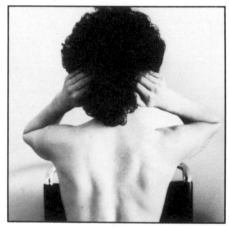

Apply firm pressure to Gall Bladder 20

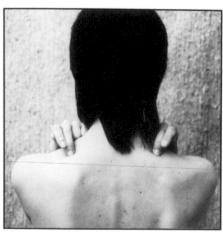

Apply firm pressure to Gall Bladder 21

LARGE INTESTINE
Acupuncture Pressure Points

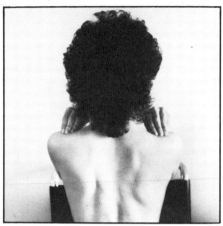

Apply firm pressure to Large intestine 16

EMOTIONALLY UPSETTING SITUATIONS

Hold the frontal eminences on the forehead for up to ten minutes. Often two or three minutes are sufficient. The posterior fontanel, (the baby's soft spot on the back of the head), corresponds to the adrenal glands, which are always in need of normalization after a traumatic event. Hold this point for 2-10 minutes, depending upon the severity of the situation. You will know when you have held both the frontal eminence points and the adrenal points a sufficient length of time, for you will suddenly realize that the problem which was so upsetting no longer seems to be disturbing your psyche. Feel for a light pulse in the correct location.

SMALL INTESTINE
Acupuncture Pressure Points

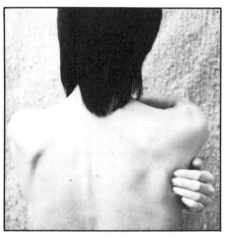

Apply firm pressure to Small intestine 11

STOMACH
Neuro-vascular Holding Points

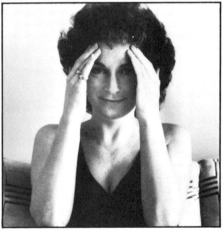

Hold the prominent bulges on your forehead (frontal eminence)

TRIPLE WARMER
Neuro-vascular Holding Point

Locate this point on the Posterior fontanel

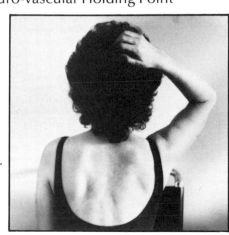

6) PRIVATE MOMENTS IN PUBLIC PLACES

Most people cope continually with some sort of nagging physical problem, be it headaches, constipation or digestive disturbances, or with a more serious matter like glaucoma, ulcers or liver or kidney malfunctioning. There are pressure points and techniques that, when implemented on a daily basis, will help to right or stabilize most conditions of ill health. Employing the correct pressure points for your condition will encourage your body's natural healing mechanism to work more effectively and quickly, and thereby speed up your recovery or stabilize your condition. Most conditions respond if you are diligent and work your points four to six times a day. This may seem like a lot of work, but it's not. When you consider how much time you spend daily taking pills or worrying needlessly about your condition, you will realize that ten to fifteen minutes spread out over a day is very little time indeed. Aim to make the use of your points a matter of habit. Schedule their use as you see fit for your lifestyle, but make it as requisite as breathing or eating. The points can also be used whenever you feel discomfort associated with your condition.

HOW TO USE THESE POINTS: Hold, massage or apply pressure to the appropriate points for your condition at least four to six times a day. If you utilize the points less than the recommended frequency, you will get slower results, although you will still experience some assistance and relief. The secret is to work the points for your condition many times daily for 1-3 minutes at a time. Frequent applications keep a constant flow of energy, blood, nutrients and lymph circulating to or through the organ in question so that the body's natural healing mechanism can function more efficiently.

If you have a condition associated with any of these pressure or massage points, you will probably find that the appropriate point will be tender or a little painful. Massage or apply pressure to the point even though it hurts. You will not harm the tissue or muscle at its location, but you will help its associated organ. You will notice as you massage or apply pressure to the point that the tenderness will lessen as your condition improves.

Whenever neuro-vascular holding points are recommended, hold the points for 1-3 minutes, four to six times a day. The neuro-lymphatic massage points should be massaged 30 seconds at a time four to six times a day. Acupuncture pressure points should receive pressure for a period of one minute.

For clarification of the following points see the Neuro-vascular Holding Points Chart on pages 148 & 149, the Neuro-lymphatic Massage Points Chart on page 46 and the Meridian Acupuncture Reference Chart on pages 38 & 39.

EYES & EARS & NOSE & TEETH

Any condition related to these organs will improve from frequent massaging of the inner edge of the humerus bone in the upper arm. Massage, very firmly, the area indicated in the photograph.

KIDNEY
Neuro-lymphatic Massage Points

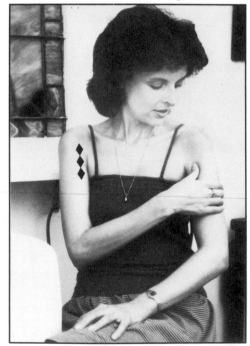

Massage firmly into the bone

GALL BLADDER CONDITIONS

Insert your middle finger into the intercostal space between the fifth and sixth ribs, which are located below the right breast or pectoralis muscle. Firmly massage the area indicated in the photograph.

GALL BLADDER
Neuro-lymphatic Massage Points

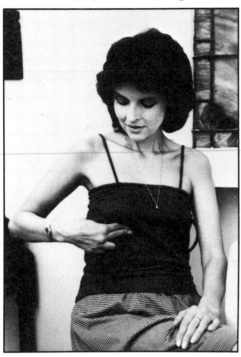

Massage firmly

REPRODUCTIVE ORGAN CONDITIONS

Apply firm thumbnail pressure or firm thumb pressure to the base of the middle fingernail at the terminal acupuncture point, and apply thumb pressure into the point at the center of the crease of the elbow. Never apply great pressure at a joint, only one that feels good and comfortable.

CIRCULATION/SEX
Acupuncture Pressure Points

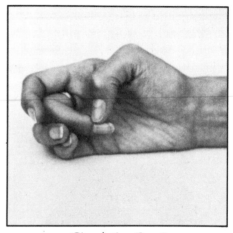

Circulation/Sex 9

CIRCULATION/SEX
Acupuncture Pressure Points

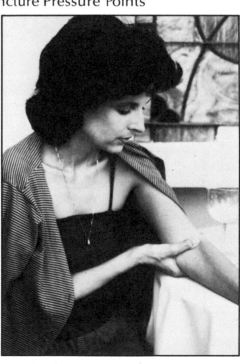

Circulation/Sex 3

ADRENAL IMBALANCE

The neuro-vascular holding point for the adrenal glands is located on the back of the head where the baby's soft spot was located. These points will help to normalize adrenal gland conditions. The lymphatic massage points for the adrenal glands are located one inch to the side of and two-and-a-half inches up from the navel. Use your middle finger, braced by the fingers on either side of it, to massage deeply into these points. It is easier to massage one side at a time when in public. These massage points should not be done before going to bed, for stimulation of the adrenal glands will keep you awake and alert. These points are useful for studying, keeping awake at concerts, driving long distances and getting a quick pick-me-up at the office.

TRIPLE WARMER
Neuro-vascular Holding Point

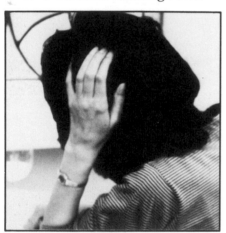

Hold lightly & feel for a pulse

Neuro-lymphatic Massage Points

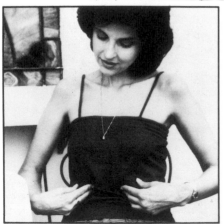

Massage firmly

BLADDER CONDITIONS

Bladder conditions caused by nervousness are greatly benefited by the frontal eminence neuro-vascular holding points. Other bladder conditions respond well to the bladder points located between the eyes, as well as the above mentioned points.

STOMACH
Neuro-vascular Holding Points

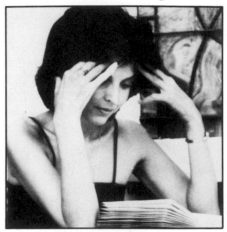

Hold lightly & feel for a pulse

BLADDER
Neuro-vascular Holding Points

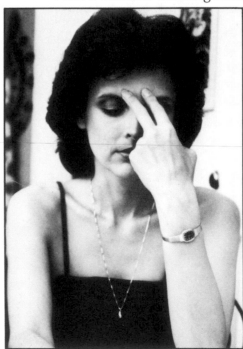

Hold lightly & feel for a pulse

SMALL INTESTINE CONDITIONS

The lymphatic massage points on the inside of the lower thigh are quite helpful for conditions of the intestinal tract and for low back pain. Use your fingers or your elbow to firmly massage the appropriate area of the thigh.

SMALL INTESTINE
Neuro-lymphatic Massage Points

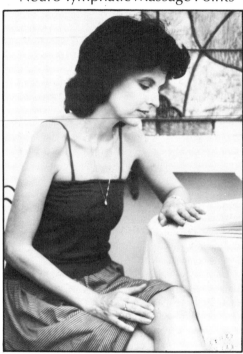

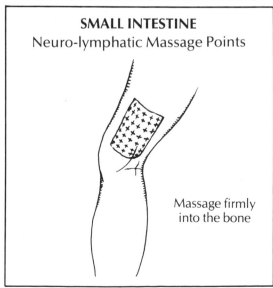

SMALL INTESTINE
Neuro-lymphatic Massage Points

Massage firmly
into the bone

STOMACH CONDITIONS

The frontal eminence neuro-vascular holding points are excellent for stomach disorders, particularly those of the nervous type. The stomach acupuncture pressure points #36 on the leg below the knee are also useful. The latter points can be done more easily in public than the frontal eminence points, although they can be done quite easily while reading at your desk.

STOMACH
Neuro-vascular Holding Points

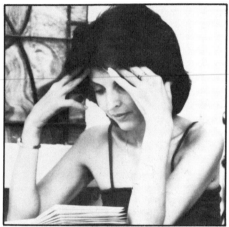

Hold lightly & feel for a pulse

STOMACH
Acupuncture Pressure Points

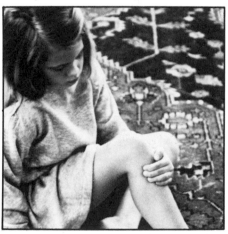

Apply firm pressure to Stomach 36

THYROID FUNCTION

Place the three middle fingers of one hand on the neuro-vascular holding points for the thyroid. The points can be held quite casually whether you are in a seated or standing position. The thyroid gland regulates the body's metabolic rate. Metabolic processes must function at the proper rate in order for all other systems to function effectively and efficiently. Hold these points gently enough to feel a light pulse with your finger tips. Do not apply pressure, for these are holding points, <u>not</u> pressure points.

TRIPLE WARMER
Neuro-vascular Holding Points

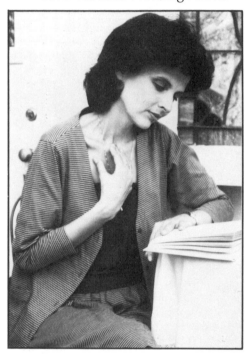

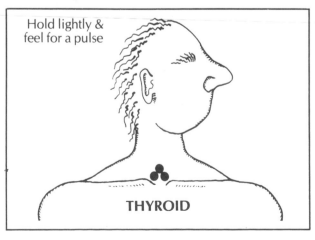

Hold lightly & feel for a pulse

THYROID

PANCREAS CONDITIONS

The neuro-vascular holding points for the pancreas are particularly beneficial to people with sugar metabolism problems. Liver points should also be done in conjunction with the pancreas points.

SPLEEN
Neuro-vascular Holding Points

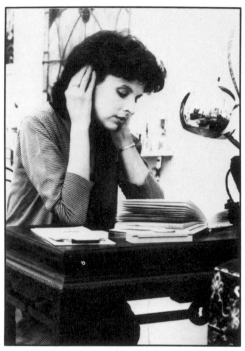

Hold Pancreas points lightly & feel for a pulse

LIVER
Neuro-vascular Holding Points

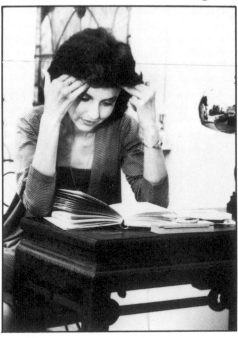

Hold lightly & feel for a pulse at the hair line

LUNG CONDITIONS

Use your thumbnail to apply firm pressure into the terminal acupuncture points for the Lung Meridian. Application of a very firm pressure also benefits these points. Do both thumbnails, unless you know specifically which lung is involved. Firm pressure into the pad of your thumb is also a good method of improving the flow of energy to the lungs.

LUNG
Acupuncture Pressure Points

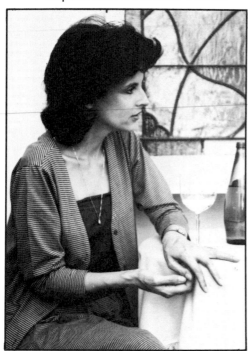

Apply firm pressure to Lung 11

LUNG
Acupuncture Pressure Points

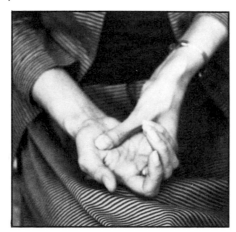

Apply firm pressure to Lung 10

LIVER POINTS

Spleen 6 on the lower inside edge of the shinbones is useful for liver disturbances. These points can also be done very inconspicuously in public. Apply firm pressure.

SPLEEN
Acupuncture Pressure Points

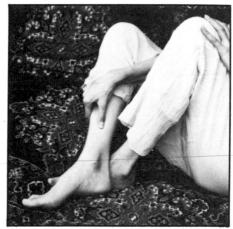

Apply firm pressure to Spleen 6

KIDNEY POINTS

Spleen 6 is beneficial to the kidneys too. Kidney 27 is another useful and easily accessible point. Use these points regularly to assist the kidneys. Don't forget to drink plenty of water. Apply firm pressure to Spleen 6 and massage Kidney 27.

KIDNEY
Neuro-lymphatic Massage Points

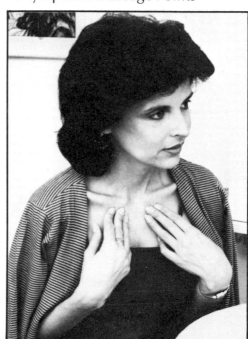

Massage firmly into the bone

HEART & CIRCULATORY CONDITIONS

Using a firm pressure, squeeze and twist the base of the fingernail for the terminal acupuncture points of the Heart and Circulation/Sex Meridians. Use your thumbnail to apply firm pressure to the points at the bases of the nails. You will know when you are on the point because it will be quite tender. Tolerate a little discomfort for a few minutes a day to avoid perhaps years of discomfort. This is a primitive form of acupuncture. It is quite effective.

HEART
Acupuncture Pressure Points

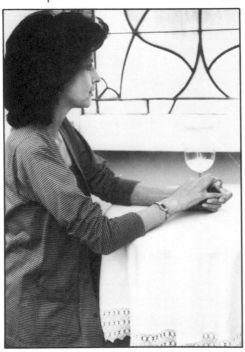

Apply firm pressure to Heart 9

CIRCULATION/SEX
Acupuncture Pressure Points

Apply firm pressure to Circulation/Sex 9

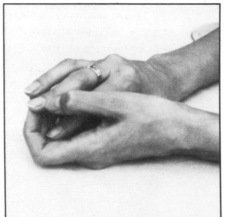

SPLEEN POINT FOR INFECTIONS

The neuro-vascular holding point for the spleen is useful for colds, flu or any infection you may contract. This point assists the immune system in its battle. Contact the holding point one-half inches above the baby soft spot on the back of the head.

SPLEEN
Neuro-vascular Holding Points

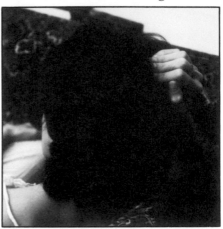

Hold lightly & feel for a pulse

CONSTIPATION

Apply firm penetrating pressure into the metacarpal bone of the index finger at the point just below the "V" where the thumb metacarpal meets the index metacarpal. This point should also be utilized while attempting to move your bowels. It is helpful to place your feet on a foot rest that is approximately three inches lower than the toilet seat. This is the correct position for efficient bowel movements. Toilet seats may be comfortable to sit on, but they are impractical because it is natural to assume a squatting position when moving the bowels.

LARGE INTESTINE
Acupuncture Pressure Points

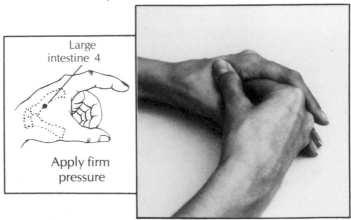

Large intestine 4

Apply firm pressure

CHAPTER VI

Factors That Increase
The Benefits of Massage

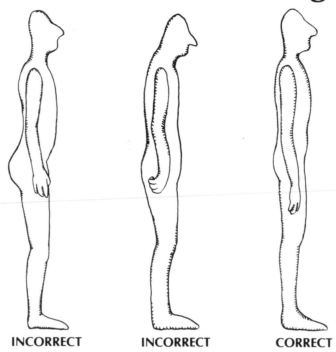

| INCORRECT | INCORRECT | CORRECT |

INTRODUCTION

In order to benefit fully and thoroughly from regular sessions of massage, you must integrate its magic into a complete program for good health. The seven sections in this chapter will introduce you to some of the necessary complements to massage therapy.

Granted, massage alone is capable of significantly upgrading your emotional and physical health and of improving or curing both chronic and acute conditions; but only a synthesis of proper diet, nutritional supplements, correct posture, regular exercise, meditation, homoeopathic medicine, general health aides and massage can achieve your long-term goal of good health. I hope the information in this chapter will stimulate your interest and set you in the right direction in your search for good health through eclectic massage.

1)POSTURE

Your posture reflects how you feel about yourself and how you see yourself in relation to other people. If you have a positive, self-confident approach to life, your posture is likely to be erect. A slumped posture, on the other hand, usually indicates a defeatist, negative attitude. The way you relate to yourself and others also determines how much your posture will succumb to the earth's constant pull of gravity. Gravity is both your enemy and your friend. Without gravity life on this planet would be impossible, but gravity also subjects you to a constant downward pull that can easily overcome you and produce an extremely exaggerated, slumped posture. As if that isn't enough, you also have to cope with postural deviations caused by other events beyond your control, like accidents, deaths, pollution, noise and all the annoyances of a modern, indifferent, technological society. It is, therefore, easy to understand why optimum posture is not so easily achieved. If you also consider that you were not taught how to walk, sit down, get up, reach or bend over, it is absolutely amazing that you're doing as well as you are. Imagine what a little correctional training could do for you!

In light of the overwhelming odds against good posture, the logical question to ask is what you can do to correct your understandable deficiencies. There is a method known as the Alexander Technique that offers a working solution to the problem. The Alexander Technique evolved over a period of ten years through concentrated effort by its originator, F. Matthias Alexander. Since the late nineteenth century, people from all walks of life have been benefiting from his discoveries. Among the more renowned people who have praised him and used his methods are Sir Charles Sherrington, John Dewey, Lilly Langtry, Professor Nikolaas Tinbergen, Aldous Huxley, Gertrude Stein's brother Leo, and George Bernard Shaw. The Alexander Technique is very popular among dancers, singers, actors and musicians, because proper posture is of utmost importance when you want to be the best in your field. For this reason, too, scientists, doctors and concerned lay people have employed the Alexander Technique. Why shouldn't each of us strive to be the best we can be?

Correct posture is basic to optimum health. If your neck is thrust forward and down, if your chest sags and your back is humped at the shoulders and arched in the lower lumbar region, how can the necessary blood, energy and nutrients reach your internal organs or muscles? Such a deformed posture weighs heavily on your internal organs, especially on your lungs, and hinders the functioning of the digestive and circulatory systems. Many conditions, including headaches, eye problems, hearing loss, digestive disturbances, chronic shoulder and neck tension, lower back pain and mental fatigue are all closely related to poor posture. Many other ailments also respond to improved posture. Contact a teacher trained in the Alexander Technique and begin lessons. You will be surprised at the number of your physical and emotional complaints that will disappear or lessen after a few lessons. Allow an Alexander teacher to reeducate you by correcting your postural habits and movements. Instructors will begin by creating an awareness of the bad habits you are now practicing and will then teach you how to correct and replace them with new postural habits and movements.

If you are interested in improving your physical and emotional lot, I very emphatically recommend that you now begin to take Alexander lessons in order to correct your postural deviations. Massage can and does improve the posture, as well as the flow of blood, nutrients and energy to internal organs and muscles. The improvement, however, is often temporary, because most people have not been sufficiently reeducated as to their abnormal holding and movement patterns. Ideally, massage therapy should come after or in conjunction with your reeducation in correct postural alignment. Don't misinterpret. Massage is always helpful, but it will have a more lasting and profound effect on your entire system if your posture is optimal.

Attempting to improve your health without correcting faulty posture is like trying to build a house on a lop-sided foundation and around a poorly constructed frame. Such a house would not do well under stress and strain. How can you, therefore, expect your body to react favorably to tension and disease with poor posture and alignment as your foundation and frame?

2) EXERCISE

Strenuous exercise is a marvelous way to lose weight, firm flabby tissue, build muscles, improve circulation, clear the lymphatic system and generally improve your health. Unfortunately, many of us are so out of shape that starting a rigorous exercise program is often disastrous. Too many people end up with more aches and pains than they had prior to their enthusiastic embarkment on a new exercise program. It's no wonder, for attempting a serious exercise program with poor alignment can only lead to injury. If your shoulders are rounded, your upper back hunched over and your lower back arched, you are no longer using the muscles of your body as you should. A body this much out of alignment cannot tolerate the demands that strenuous exercise puts on the skeletal and muscular systems. Attempting to do too much too soon and choosing the wrong kind of exercise for your body type are two other common reasons why exercise often proves to be detrimental rather than beneficial. So, before you embark on an exercise program, treat yourself first to a series of Alexander lessons. Then choose the proper form of exercise for your body type and lifestyle.

If you feel that your posture is quite good, as I did, you will be surprised how much more Alexander lessons can teach you about the many subtle adjustments and significant changes necessary for your body to achieve optimum posture and health. During and after your lessons you will experience a new-found freedom of movement and grace, as well as a significant improvement in your emotional equilibrium.

Before I suggest some preferred types of exercises, allow me to say a few words about jogging, our nation's favorite way to exercise. Jogging can work wonderfully to tone your body, strengthen your muscles and improve your vascular system. It can also do a lot of harm. Most people out there jogging are not fit for it. Unless your body is lithe and your posture close to perfect, you should forget about running your body to health. People with large bones, stalky builds, poor posture, excess weight or large breasts should not be jogging. Every step you take jars your entire spinal column and all the joints in your legs. In addition, your internal organs also take quite a beating on each successive impact. The medical profession is making millions of dollars annually on self-inflicted injuries related to jogging, not to mention injuries resulting from accidents with moving vehicles. Jogging on concrete is absolutely out of the question for the above-mentioned reasons. Jogging in or near traffic and inhaling those carbon-monoxide fumes is totally ridiculous. Unless you can run on a wooden track or on turf in a park or in the country, forget it. You'd probably be better off not running at all.

An excellent substitute for jogging is rebounding on a small trampoline. Set up your trampoline near an open window or outdoors. Then jog, kick, twist and jump to your heart's content, without experiencing any of the negative side-effects of jogging. Rebounding is easy to do, and it exercises every muscle and strengthens every cell in your body. Most important, trampolining is fun, and all you need is ten minutes twice a day to make it profitable exercise. Any more than ten minutes at a time does not significantly increase the benefits. Rebound first thing in the morning to get your adrenal glands and circulation going for the whole day. Rebound before meals to curb your appetite. Rebound while watching television. Rebound if you're feeling tired. Rebound any time at all. In a matter of three days you will be hooked and loving it. Rebounding is safe. It's economical, as a trampoline is a one-time investment. It's not time-consuming, and it strengthens and tones your entire body. Besides all that, it's lots of FUN.

There are many different ways to exercise, but I am only going to recommend exercises that develop both sides of your body equally. That leaves out tennis, handball, racketball, baseball and the like, because such sports demand the use of one side of the body more than the other. They thus encourage unnatural tension and strain on the skeletal and muscular systems. Instead, consider exercises like jogging on turf or wooden track, very fast walking with arms swinging freely, trampolining, yoga, Tai Chi Chuan, roller-skating, swimming, body-building or cross-country skiing.

Yoga and Tai Chi Chuan are excellent for toning and stretching muscles, for improving balance and for effecting relaxation, but neither do as much for the vascular system as more active forms of exercise. Therefore, if you practice yoga or Tai Chi Chuan daily, you would do well also to trampoline or practice any of the other suggested types of exercise.

Exercise is necessary, though usually difficult for most of us to do regularly. If you haven't found a form of exercise that comes to you easily, consider trampolining. Whatever you choose, before you pursue it, remember to get your postural problems corrected, if possible, with an Alexander teacher.

Massage, a passive form of exercise, affects our system in much the same way as active, willful forms of exercise. The effects are not as profound, but circulation, lymph flow and muscle tone do improve. Massage can even exercise and free tension from the joints of the body through the use of mechanotherapy techniques. Mechanotherapy can be passive, in which case the therapist does the joint manipulation; active, in which case the receiver willfully puts the joints through the range of motion; or resisted, in which case the massage therapist or the receiver resists the movements. Unless a person is extremely ill or disabled, massage cannot serve as a substitute for exercise. It can, however, complement and enhance the beneficial effects of an exercise program. Because regular exercise lowers tension levels and generally improves body functions, the massage therapist can reach deep-seated tensions rather than superficial ones.

3)DIET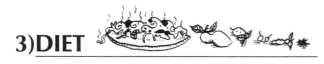

A young woman of twenty-four once came to me for massage with complaints of extreme fatigue, depression, lack of concentration, failing vision, poor digestion, inability to sleep, poor balance and a general lack of interest in everything from her work to intimate dinner dates. I immediately suspected that she needed more than massage, so I asked her what constituted her diet on an average day. She proceeded to tell me that she had two cups of coffee with sugar and a pastry for breakfast; a coke and a roast beef sandwich on a white roll with mayonnaise, but no lettuce, for lunch; and cookies with a glass of milk for dinner, because she was too tired to cook for herself. This was her daily diet. No fruit, no vegetables, no whole grains and lots of sugar. I very quickly explained to her that massage would be of no use to her, unless she was willing to improve her diet.

You are what you eat, or don't eat, and this young woman was a perfect example of what you are because of what you do or don't eat. Your diet directly affects your skeletal, muscular, nervous, circulatory, respiratory, digestive, integumentary (skin), urinary and endocrine systems. If your body does not receive the nutrients needed to maintain its complicated body processes, you will begin experiencing maladies of all types: first fatigue, then aches and pains, then depression, and finally disease. Fortunately, this young woman followed a rejuvenation diet consisting of plenty of fruits, vegetables, whole grains and high quality protein, so that she regained her health before the disease stage set in. Not so fortunately, many people never find their way to a practitioner who is able to offer them correct advice or guidance.

There is a growing number of doctors, professionals and lay people who stand in agreement with the accumulating scientific proof that we are indeed what we do or don't eat. Unfortunately, many people, including doctors, scientists and professionals, refuse to accept this obvious fact. Why is it so difficult for the intelligent, well-educated mind to accept the obvious? Few people would fuel their car with inferior gas or oil and expect it to run efficiently. How can your body operate efficiently on such inferior foods as soda, coffee, candy and refined or processed foods? Why don't people see the correlation?

The ability to accept change freely is the underlying problem. It seems to be fundamental to human nature to resist change as long as possible. Throughout human history many famous scientists and doctors have confronted the world with revolutionary ideas, only to find themselves and their ideas ignored or denounced as fanatical or heretical. Linus Pauling is a perfect example. He fought against the system in his attempt to get the medical community to recognize the wonders of Vitamin C. He finally won a Nobel prize for his work, and then discovered that his efforts were recognized on paper only. One hopes the time has come to stop resisting the facts. Diet affects our bodies and minds.

Apart from resisting change, there are other reasons why people won't or can't accept the obvious correlation between diet and health. Advertising campaigns, which are backed by big industry, and personal as well as cultural habits also prevent people from accepting the blatantly obvious. Big industry and advertising companies have overwhelmingly succeeded in brainwashing the vast majority of the public into believing that refined and processed foods are equal to or even superior in quality to their natural counterparts. Cultural conditioning and personal habits, added to the successful brainwashing campaigns by manufacturers and producers, have continually foiled the necessary changes in attitude toward diet and nutrition.

How did refined, processed and injected food arrive on the market? Originally, I believe, the intention of the farmers, cattle breeders, fowl raisers and manufacturers were at least partially honorable. They wanted as much fresh, top-quality food to reach the public as possible. They also liked the ideas of preservatives, refining and artificial fertilization, largely because they improved profits. There's nothing wrong with wanting to improve profits, as long as you are producing a quality product. When all these changes and so-called improvements were initially made, few people realized how dangerous these chemicals and refining processes were. The original laboratory tests, if any, were performed on a short-term basis. Thus, the extent of the dangers of chemical additives and refining processes were relatively unknown, not only to the general public, but also to those directly involved with the production and preparation of food. By the time most people became aware of the hazards to their health, it was too late to reverse the process. As so much money had been invested in these new ideas, it was financially impractical to stop midstream and lose fortunes. Most of our providers have chosen to continue this trend without caring about the results, or perhaps they are blindly hoping that somehow it will all work out.

Refined, processed, injected and artificially fertilized foods are a relatively new addition to our diets, but they have been thoroughly accepted by most people, because of and with no thanks to heavily financed advertising campaigns.

The refining and processing of foods took hold in the early part of the twentieth century. Before then, most of our ancestors ate whole grains and unadulterated foods that had been organically fertilized.

Why alter a perfectly acceptable food to a less acceptable one? Refining whole grains by removing those parts that contain oil insures fresh grains and bakery goods, but it also makes for nutritiously inferior products. Adding preservatives, artificial color and flavor to foods extends their shelf life and increases their visual appeal. These processes mask the inferiority of the food. Also the chemicals over-burden the liver. It is far better to provide proper refrigeration for foods than to strip them of their life-giving properties and to mask the unacceptable end-product with artificial color and flavor.

Fertilization of the crops you consume is another important factor to consider when the nutrient content of a food is at question. Synthetic fertilizers provide a faster and easier way to ensure larger yields and more visually appealing crops than do organic fertilizers, but the food you eat is ultimately less nutritious. Synthetic fertilizers are leeches to the soil. They yield inferior crops, because many of the minerals that would be available in organically fertilized soils are simply not present in synthetically fertilized soil.

What is the end-result of the refining and artificial fertilization that our crops and grains undergo? The foods we consume are so depleted of their natural nutrients that the vast majority of people who shop in supermarkets are suffering from a wide variety of subclinical malnutrition symptoms. The medical profession refuses to acknowledge this fact, although more and more doctors are slowly beginning to recognize the importance of the quality of the food you consume. Producers and manufacturers are slowly, or perhaps quickly, starving and/or poisoning us with nutrient-deficient crops that are also heavily laden with dangerous chemical additives.

It is impossible to receive optimum nutrition from refined and processed foods. Chemically leeched soils diminish the nutrients we receive in our vegetables, fruits and grains. Over-burdening the land, either by not rotating crops regularly or by not planting rotation crops to replenish the soil, further reduces the available organic compounds in our food. Harvesting unripe vegetables and fruit diminishes still more the total of vitamins and minerals available to our bodies to metabolize. Crops that are picked green are never as nutritious as those ripened on the vine, for they have not had the time necessary to receive their full share of nutrients from the soil.

Transportation and storage further complicate matters. Many shipping and storage companies lack the refrigeration necessary to keep the products fresh and thus to ensure their food values. Retail dealers often add insult to injury by not providing refrigeration for the display of their fresh produce. Many foods lose at least 50% of certain vitamins in the twenty-four to forty-eight hour period after harvesting.

Add to all these commercial practices the common household practice of overcooking foods, as well as that of keeping fruits and vegetables at room temperature for days prior to their consumption, and it should be startlingly clear that it's difficult, if not impossible, to get the nutrients your body needs from the food you eat. Considering all the possibilities for the food you purchase to lose nutrients valuable to you, how many of those essential nutrients do you suppose are still actually in the fruits and vegetables you eat? Certainly not enough to maintain a sound, healthy, happy body and mind.

"But, statistics indicate the people live much longer today than they ever have before, so how bad can our diet be?" Statements like this, which defend the modern diet, may at first seem sound, but statistics rarely mean what they appear to say. Although government statistics indicate that life expectancy today is much longer than it ever was before, these statistics are deceptive. True, infant mortality has dropped. So have deaths due to accidents because of improved emergency medical care. Heart attacks do not now result in death as often as they did in the past because of advances in medical technology. Nor do very many of us in the modern age suffer the deleterious effects of working twelve to sixteen hours a day in subhuman factory conditions, and

most of us are fortunate enough to live in well-heated homes that protect us from fatal illnesses related to cold and dampness. Certainly we are living longer, but not because of our wonderful diet. Modern technology, not an optimum diet, has managed to save many lives and lengthen life expectancy.

From farm to marketplace to household, the insults to our foods are endless. Flesh foods, no less than fruits and vegetables, have been drastically altered by modern practices. Breeders of fowl and cattle today widely and commonly use female hormones to fatten up their animals and to increase their profits. Profits, however, are not the only things increasing. The size of men's hips and breasts are also increasing, and the use of female hormones has considerably upped the incidence of acne in both men and women. Also, antibiotics which are now regularly used to protect fowl and cattle from sickness adversely affect the consumer. The small doses of antibiotic drugs in the flesh foods some people constantly consume have undermined and weakened their immune systems, and thus broken down their resistance to illness and disease. What is the end result of all the additives, hormones, antibiotics and refining processes? Fatigue, aches and pains, depression, poor overall health and a significant rise in illness and disease.

What can you do to improve your eating habits and to avoid all these hazards? Is there a diet that will offer you physical well-being, good mental health and a happy psychological state? Yes, there is, and it is one that has worked for many.

Start by reverting to unrefined, unprocessed, naturally fertilized and additive-free foods. Also eliminate all beef and pork products, including such processed meats as salami, bologna, sausages and ham. Already you will be well on your way to a healthy diet. Instead of buying commercial chicken, seek out a source for fowl that is free of hormones and antibiotics. Consume a variety of fresh fish. Make NO soda, NO fried foods, NO refined sugars and NO salt your new rules to live by. The occasional use of sun-dried sea salt is fine, by the way. Forget about canned or frozen vegetables and fruit, and consume only whole grain noodles, crackers, breads and desserts. No more white rice, either, I'm afraid, for it's brown rice from now on. Undercook rather than overcook your food, and seventy to eighty percent of your food should be eaten raw. Whenever possible, consume organically grown food, because their soils, composted naturally, are free of chemicals and supply the fruits and vegetables and you with more nutrients. Finally, don't fry. The only acceptable methods of cooking are boiling, baking, steaming, and for soups, simmering.

It sounds easy, doesn't it? It's not, however, quite as easy as I'd like. I've just summarized in a few sentences the major changes you need in your diet, but change, as I mentioned earlier, does not come easily for the majority of us. These dietary changes will mean not only eating different foods but also shopping in different stores, particularly health food stores. Shop the supermarkets for toilet paper, tissues and paper towels, as well as for the occasional health food items they sometimes stock, but you'll have to buy most of your new food staples at a health food store. Also, start frequenting health food restaurants, as the foods they serve generally conform to the requirements of your new diet. Although these changes may sound overwhelming to you, once you begin to implement them, your newly found awareness of better health will encourage you to continue your new program.

Some health professionals believe that all illness and disease can be cured or controlled through optimal diet and supplemental nutrition. When we know all there is to know about nutritional therapy, we might well say that these professionals marched ahead of their times and saw beyond all current medical knowledge. Chances are, however, there will always be some diseases that cannot be cured through diet and nutritional therapy alone. Since I am a skeptic, I would state that only most of our illnesses and diseases can be controlled or cured through proper diet and nutrition; these must be supplemented further with proper exercise, stress control, correct homoeopathic preparations and Alexander lessons or chiropractics to effect optimum structural alignment and posture. Once you begin to supply your body daily with the essential nutrients needed to carry on its complex metabolic functions and begin to attend regularly to the other essential components for good health, your body will begin to perform efficiently for you.

The following pages summarize the major food categories and indicate the preferable choices in each of them. Recommendations are also made as to how many times daily each of the food types should be consumed. Following the information on the major types of foods is a section on food combining, which includes some sample suggestions for snacks. Snacks are preferable to large meals, and when you have mastered the food combining rules, you will be confident enough to create varied, proper and healthful snacks of your own.

PROTEIN *(3 or 4 servings daily)*

EGGS–fertile, no hormones or antibiotics, from free-running flocks (raw, soft or hard-boiled, poached, baked)
TOFU–organically grown, no preservatives, unpasteurized (raw, steamed, baked, broiled, simmered in soups)
TEMPEH–organically grown, no preservatives (raw, steamed, baked, broiled, simmered in soups)
CHICKEN–no hormones or antibiotics, free-running flocks (baked, broiled)
FISH–fresh only, variety is important so consider: fresh vs. salt water, low vs. high fat, small vs. large (broiled, baked, steamed or raw)
MILK–certified raw *only*
BUTTERMILK–salt-free
YOGHURT–live cultures, plain, sugar-free
KEFIR–preferably plain
COTTAGE CHEESE–low fat, salt-free, no sugar (as often as you like)
CHEESE–raw milk, salt-free, no artificial color once a week if there is no problem with constipation or mucous

FRESH VEGETABLES (3 or 4 colors daily)

— preferably raw in a salad or lightly steamed
BEAN SPROUTS—daily
SEAWEED—nori and dulse seem to be the most enjoyable raw—hiziki is wonderful cooked
LETTUCE—the darker the lettuce, the richer in vitamins and minerals, e.g. romaine
ROOT VEGETABLES—organically grown, unradiated
BROCCOLI—no yellow buds, dark green only
any other vegetable you enjoy

FRESH FRUIT (1 or 2 daily)

APPLES • PEARS • GRAPES • BANANAS •
CITRUS FRUITS—do not consume more than twice weekly or you risk becoming too alkaline
any other fruit you enjoy

DRIED FRUIT (occasionally)

—limit quantity because of the high natural sugar content
—no sugar or honey dipped fruit
—buy only unsulphured fruit
RAISINS • APRICOTS • FIGS
any other dried fruit you enjoy, but concentrate on the above as they are richest in minerals.

FRESH JUICES (as desired)

Fruit and vegetable juices are a highly concentrated food. Do not drink more than four ounces of any fresh juice at one time, because juice is too concentrated for the liver. Swish or "chew" the juice in your mouth for a few seconds before swallowing, so your body knows what's coming down. Consume all juices, except for fresh apple cider, immediately after squeezing in order to avoid the harmful effects of oxidization. Drinking moderate amounts of fresh juices can be beneficial to your health. Do not defeat your purpose by drinking too many juices or by drinking oxidized juices. Brown carrot juice is an example of oxidized juice. Fresh carrot juice is bright orange. Do not drink too many citrus fruit juices.

LEGUMES (daily)

—consume with rice as an alternative to animal protein
—consume legumes in combination with rice or grains in order to obtain a complete protein
KIDNEY • BLACK-EYED PEAS • PINTO •
CHICK PEAS • GREEN or YELLOW SPLIT or WHOLE PEAS • LENTILS
PEANUTS

NUTS (daily)

(refrigerate—raw only)
ALMONDS (the preferred nut)
FILBERTS • WALNUTS •
NO CASHEWS—cashews are almost always rancid; if you want the taste of raw cashews, eat *raw* cashew butter

SEEDS (daily)

(refrigerate—raw only)
SUNFLOWER • PUMPKIN •
SESAME—use raw sesame butter or tahini instead of the seeds: As most people do not thoroughly chew the seeds, they pass through the digestive tract undigested

RICE (daily)

BROWN • WILD RICE

GRAINS (daily)

—refrigerate ground grains because the natural oils go rancid very quickly
—variety is important
BUCKWHEAT • WHOLE WHEAT • MILLET •
CORN • RYE • OATS
any other whole grain you enjoy

BREAD (daily)

DO NOT REFRIGERATE as moisture is pulled out of bread faster when it is refrigerated; store in a cool dark place.

MULTIGRAIN BREADS

WHOLE WHEAT—be sure label reads "whole wheat," not "wheat flour"

CORN

RYE—beware of commercial rye breads; read the label for ingredients

any other whole grain bread you enjoy
(not pumpernickel, unless you are certain of
all the ingredients)

CRACKERS (as desired)

Whole grain only—salt-free, sea salt occasionally—no shortening or hydrogenated oils—no sugar—rice cakes are an interesting alternative to crackers

NOODLES (as desired)

There are many different types of noodles now on the health food market. Be sure the label specifies *whole* wheat noodles, NOT wheat noodles. Even your children will love them. Spirulina noodles and soya noodles enhance the protein content of your meals.

VEGETABLE OILS (daily)

—refrigerate
—variety is important
—consume only mechanically pressed, unrefined, unfiltered oils that are free of solvents, bleaches, dyes and preservatives
SESAME • SAFFLOWER • SUNFLOWER
any other oil you enjoy

ANIMAL FATS (occasionally)

SWEET RAW BUTTER • SOUR CREAM—salt-free
HEAVY CREAM—not ultrapasteurized

SALAD DRESSING (as desired)

—homemade preparations are preferable
—use only unprocessed oils
—use apple-cider vinegar, not white vinegar
—fresh lemon juice is an excellent alternative to apple-cider vinegar

MISCELLANEOUS

—tamari instead of soy sauce
—miso for broth base, be sure it contains sea salt, NOT table salt
—tekka is a condiment for rice, noodles or steamed vegetables (sprinkle over food just prior to serving)

SPICES

The first three listed are beneficial to your health Add to your food after it is cooked in order to maintain the beneficial qualities
GARLIC • CAYENNE • GINGER • CURRY
any other spice you enjoy
use moderately

HERBS

DILL • PARSLEY • THYME • TARRAGON
OREGANO
any other herb you enjoy

SWEETENERS

HONEY—tupelo honey metabolizes more slowly than other honey, and therefore is preferable
BLACKSTRAP MOLASSES • PURE MAPLE SYRUP • MALT

WATER *(6-8 glasses daily)*

—20 minutes before meals or 1 1/2-2 hours after a meal, so digestive juices are not diluted
—variety is important; each water has different mineral concentrations
—glass bottles are preferable to plastic, because the plastic bleeds into the water
PERRIER • EVIAN • MOUNTAIN VALLEY
any other reputable bottled water

FOOD COMBINING

WHAT IS FOOD COMBINING?

Food combining perhaps defines itself, but eating foods from the various major categories in a combination that can be easily digested requires method. It also requires alteration of common eating habits. Rather than eating three large meals a day, you will be enjoying frequent small snacks. Your body will be able to utilize all the calories and nutrients that it needs. Eat 4 to 6 small snacks daily. Eat every 3 or 4 hours. Drink water 20 to 30 minutes before each snack.

WHY FOOD COMBINING

* You will lose weight safely and maintain your proper body weight

* Your general health will improve

* You will experience more energy

* Your digestive system will not be overworked

* You will experience relief from gas, belching and bloating

* Your elimination will become more regular

* Your complexion will improve

WHAT ARE THE BASIC RULES?

1) Fruits and vegetables must be consumed at different snacks.
2) Non-starchy vegetables combine best with proteins or starches.
3) Starchy root vegetables combine best with non-starchy vegetables or legumes.
4) Proteins and sweets don't mix, therefore no sweet & sour dishes.
5) Animal protein and starch don't mix, therefore no flesh foods with potatoes, bread, noodles, rice, etc.
6) Raw milk or cultured milk products must be consumed alone or only with acid fruits, e.g. berries, oranges, pineapples, grapes.
7) Melons are best eaten alone. Some people find that melon in a fresh fruit salad digests easily. If you don't bloat and don't experience gas, belching or fatigue, enjoy melon in fruit salad.
8) Cereals and grains combine best with vegetables or legumes.
9) Oils and fats combine best with green and non-starchy vegetables. Exception: cream & berries combine well.
10) Legumes, beans and peas combine best with vegetables, rice or grains.
11) Seeds and nuts should be consumed separately. Most people seem to digest seeds and nuts together quite well. If you do not experience difficulty when you eat these two together, feel free to do so.

The complete rules for food combining get slightly more complicated, but these are the combinations most important to your awareness and for your attention.

Now that you know the healthful benefits of food combining and its basic rules, the next step is to implement the rules and incorporate food combining into your daily life. It may sound easy, but it involves undoing years of conditioning. From experience I have found that most people are simply at a loss when it comes to combining foods properly. It takes a while to learn how to prepare healthful, appetizing snacks. Old habits are so overpowering that most people simply don't know what to eat, unless it's what they're accustomed to preparing and serving. I have assembled some of my favorite snacks for you, so you will have something to work with until you feel confident enough to create some exciting new snacks of your own.

But first, one word about dessert is necessary. If you really crave something sweet once in a while, the thing to have is a sweet snack. Any sweet snack, other than fresh fruit, is automatically going to be a cheat, so don't make matters worse by combining it with something else. There is one exception, however, and that's a salad. Follow your sweet snack with a healthy green salad. The minerals in the salad greens will help your body to cope with the high dose of sugar. Limit your sweet treats to goodies purchased from your local health food store. Read the labels on all sweets you purchase, however, as even health food stores sell questionable products. If you have time to bake your own sweets, do so, because only then can you be absolutely certain of the purity of the ingredients. Use only unrefined and unprocessed foods in the preparation of your sweet treats, and do not consume them too often. Unless you have been instructed by your holistic physician to avoid all sweets, occasional whole grain, unrefined sweet treats will not harm you.

Here, then, are some of my favorite snacks:

1) Yoghurt or salt-free buttermilk or Kefir with fresh berries
2) Mixed nuts and a 3-4 color salad.
3) Pumpkin and sunflower seeds with a 3- color salad
4) Fish and a 3- color salad
5) Chicken or fish and steamed vegetables, 3 colors
6) Rice and beans with salad
7) Steamed vegetables with rice and beans
8) Whole grain bread, bagel or muffin with peanut butter and bean sprouts
9) Brown rice or whole wheat noodles covered with steamed vegetables, tofu cubes and tahini sauce*
10) Soft-boiled eggs served with finely chopped, steamed mixed vegetables seasoned with Vegit and/or cayenne
11) Soft-boiled eggs served with fresh, chopped alfalfa sprouts seasoned with Vegit and/or cayenne, or herbs of your choice

12) Salt-free cottage cheese with 3-color vegetable salad
13) Slices of tofu marinated in fresh lemon juice, tamari and ginger served with a small bowl of brown rice or noodles covered with tahini sauce.* A salad or steamed vegetables will compliment the tofu and rice.
14) Noodles topped with blended tofu, tahini, tamari and spices of your choice. Garnish with finely chopped scallions and grated carrots.
15) Noodles and fake tomato sauce. Blend steamed carrots, squash , onions and tofu. Season with oregano for an Italian touch or with curry and cardamon for a spicy Indian taste. Stir in lightly steamed dark green vegies just prior to serving for color effect. Serve with a salad.

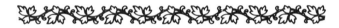

*TAHINI SAUCE

—1/2 jar raw sesame tahini
—tamari to taste
—cayenne to taste and/or garlic
—enough water to make into a medium-thick sauce
—blend in a blender
—do not cook; pour directly over hot food

Some healthful foods may have been unintentionally omitted. Eat them if they are whole, unrefined and free of additives. Remember, variety is of utmost importance. A mono-diet can get boring and won't supply all the nutrients you need in order to be healthy.

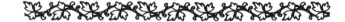

4) SUPPLEMENTAL NUTRITION

Proper eating habits cannot always guarantee you the optimum dietary health you seek. You, like many others, may have greater needs for one or more nutrients than do most people. Your job may expose you to toxins or stresses that increase your vitamin and mineral requirements. Emotional problems drain your body and increase its need for certain nutrients. Fluoridated water and air pollution also rob the body of essential minerals and vitamins. Finally, a hereditary predisposition to a particular disease will increase your need for certain nutrients.

It is possible to obtain the extra nutrients you require either by taking supplements or by eating more of the foods that are high in the needed minerals and vitamins. The parts of the body listed below have been known to respond to particular nutrients and foods. Consult a qualified nutritionist or a holistically oriented physician to determine the exact amount of any nutrient you need.

PART OF BODY	VITAMINS	MINERALS	FOODS
Hair (color)	A, B-Complex, C (PABA)	Sulphur Iodine Copper	protein, nuts, citrus fruit, fish liver oil, dark leafy greens, carrots, brewer's yeast
Nails	A, B-Complex	Sulphur Iron Calcium	protein, fish liver oil, yeast, raisins, yoghurt
Ear Infections	A, B-Complex E		protein, citrus fruit, fish liver oil
Teeth & Gums	A, C, D	Calcium Magnesium Phosphorus Iron	leafy green vegetables, protein, fresh fruit, whole grain bread
Mucous Membranes (nose, lungs, intestines, etc.)	A		fish liver oils
Thyroid		Iodine	seaweed & ocean fish
Lungs	A, D, E, C	Iron	fish liver oil, organ meats, wheat germ oil, citrus fruit, eggs, blackstrap molasses, green leafy vegetables
Heart	E Thiamine	Calcium Phosphorous Potassium	brewer's yeast, wheat germ, oil, yoghurt, eggs, seeds, nuts, whole grains, leafy green vegetables, bananas
Liver	A, D, E, B-Complex		protein, fish liver oil, brewer's yeast, wheat germ oil, dark green vegetables, organic chicken livers

PART OF BODY	VITAMINS	MINERALS	FOODS
Stomach	B-Complex (Niacin)		brewer's yeast
Gall Bladder (stones)	A, D, E B-Complex		protein, fish liver oil, wheat germ oil, green leafy vegetables
Kidney (stones)		Magnesium	apples, almonds, figs, leafy green vegetables
Bladder (cystitis)	A, C, E B-Complex		fish liver oil, brewer's yeast, citrus fruit, wheat germ oil
Large Intestines (constipation)	A, C, B-Complex		water (6-8 glasses per day), 2-3 tbspns. coarse bran, fish liver oil, brewer's yeast, citrus fruit
Diarrhea	Increase all vitamins & minerals to compensate for loss of nutrients		low fiber, protein, fish liver oil, brewer's yeast, citrus fruit, bananas
Reproductive & Sexual Organs	E B-Complex (folic acid)	Iron Zinc (males) Iodine	wheat germ oil, brewer's yeast, raisins, eggs, sunflower seeds, fish & poultry, mushrooms, seaweed
Pancreas (diabetes)	C, A	Zinc Chromium Manganese	citrus fruit, fish liver oil, seeds & nuts, brewer's yeast, green leafy vegetables
Skin (dry)	A, D B-Complex		fish liver oil, protein, raisins, yoghurt, brewer's yeast
Leg Cramps	E	Calcium & Magnesium	wheat germ oil, yoghurt, molasses, nuts, green leafy vegetables

IMPORTANT: Suck on all your vitamin and mineral supplements until your mouth fills with saliva. When this occurs, your body has been prepared for what is on its way down. Your assimilation will be improved if you follow these instructions.

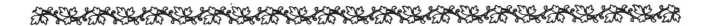

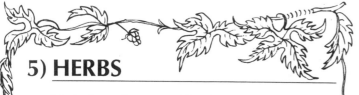

5) HERBS

Herbs have been used by doctors, medicine men, witches and lay people since the beginning of time. Rich or poor, wise or uneducated, all alike have benefited from the healing qualities of herbs. Even the Bible states that herbs are to be our medicine. Today, in our age of modern medicine, many people are reverting to the use of herbs to cure or control disease, because herbs actually cure the cause of the disease, rather than merely masking the symptoms, and also because herbs, unlike drugs, rarely have any harmful side-effects.

Herbs act as catalysts within our body. As such, they help improve the body's own natural healing mechanism. Herbs can calm as well as stimulate. They can relieve pain, aid digestion, restore consciousness, raise or lower blood pressure, beautify the skin, rejuvenate internal organ functions, relieve spasms, act as an astringent, cure diarrhea or constipation, and heal wounds.

Store herbs in airtight, dark glass or tin containers away from the light, heat and dampness. Buy small quantities from shops that have a good turnover and keep herbs for only one year.

To make an infusion or herbal tea, use one-half to one ounce of the herb to one pint of water. Bring the water to a boil, then turn off the heat and pour boiling water over the herb. Cover and steep for ten minutes. Use only glass, enamel or porcelain pots. Drink the infusion, one mouthful at a time, throughout the day. Drink the tea cool or lukewarm, unless you wish to induce sweating, as in the case of a cold.

There are many books on the market that discuss herbs, their uses and methods of preparation. *The Herb Book* by John Lust and *Back to Eden* by Jethro Kloss are considered classics in the field.

Homoeopathic preparations stimulate the body's natural healing mechanism and, unlike herbal medicine, contain substances other than herbs. The doses of these preparations are minute highly stimulating. The strength is not, however, directly related to the herb in its crude form but rather to a dynamic power derived from that herb. Consult a Homoeopathic physician for the most efficient utilization of these herbal preparations.

ACNE—dandelion, chaparral, sassafras

ADRENALS—capsicum

ANEMIA—dandelion, comfrey

BLADDER—dandelion, chamomile, comfrey, uva ursi

CIRCULATION—chickweed, capsicum, mistletoe

COLDS—comfrey, licorice, chamomile (drink or use as a vapor bath)

EYESTRAIN—eyebright (drink and use as an eye wash)

GAS PAINS—catnip, thyme, ginger

GALL BLADDER—dandelion, yellow dock

HEART—sedative: mistletoe
stimulant: wood betony, capsicum

HEMORRHOIDS—uva ursi

KIDNEY—chamomile, dandelion, comfrey, uva ursi

HIGH BLOOD PRESSURE—capsicum, passion flower

INFECTIONS—golden seal, rose hips

INSOMNIA—passion flower, german chamomile

LARGE INTESTINES—constipation: chickweed
diarrhea: comfrey, peppermint, thyme

LIVER—dandelion, uva ursi, hops

LOW BLOOD PRESSURE—dandelion

LUNGS—comfrey, thyme, chickweed, fenugreek

MENOPAUSE—black cohosh, hops

PANCREAS—dandelion, fenugreek

SEXUAL & REPRODUCTIVE ORGANS—

♀ ovaries: chamomile
general: red raspberry

♂ prostate: golden seal
urethra: golden seal

SORE THROAT—ginger (suck on a piece), golden seal

SINUS—golden seal

SPLEEN—chamomile, dandelion, uva ursi

STOMACH—comfrey, chamomile, fenugreek, ginger, lobelia

TENSION—mistletoe, passion flower, chamomile, valerian

TOOTHACHE—chamomile (hold in mouth around tooth)

TONIC—licorice, chamomile, dandelion

VITALITY—

♀ ginseng, licorice

♂ Gotu Kola, licorice

6)MEDITATION

Meditation is a very beneficial practice for all people. It can give you clarity of thought, free you from excessive tensions, improve physiological as well as psychological health and yield a more fulfilling spiritual awareness. Meditation is particularly healthful to high-strung, very active individuals who need a time once or twice a day to stop and get in touch with themselves and everything around them. Although such individuals may find it difficult to stop racing and unwind enough to meditate, it is possible with repeated practice. The rewards will prove great enough to merit the initial effort. It appears that the more a person needs meditation, the more difficult it is to find the time to achieve this state of mind.

If meditation seems to you too inextricably tied up with gurus and devotees, don't be discouraged. It is possible to learn the skill from such people and then take it home for your own personal use. On occasion you may need to return to your teacher in order to refresh your skill, but you can remain aloof from the traditional and ritualistic aspects of these institutions if you so desire.

There are many different types of meditation. I am not about to say that one is better than the next. Whichever works for you is the best for you. Transcendental Meditation is one of the more common and easily located schools of meditation. Because many articles have been written on the benefits of Transcendental Meditation in prestigious scientific journals, it is perhaps the best-known to the general public. This does not mean, however, that is the best form of meditation. Other types of meditation, like those, for example, that do not use a mantra but instead focus on a shape or color, can achieve good results if they are practiced correctly. The key is to give your all to the technique of your choice. Be patient and you will be rewarded.

Meditation and massage go hand in hand. The relaxed state of awareness achieved through meditation can be called upon when receiving a massage and can enhance its benefits. Furthermore, a person who practices meditation regularly will come to the massage therapist with less tension. The therapist will thus be able to reach deeper into the essence of the subject, instead of having to work with all the tensions that accumulate from week to week. In other words, greater and deeper releases will be achieved to provide more fulfillment and rewards for both the therapist and the receiver.

7)GENERAL AIDS

There are many general health aids that can be purchased from both health food stores and department stores. These devices can be used in your home to improve your general health. Some are inexpensive and others are quite the opposite, but they are all worthwhile investments. This section describes some of the more common and popular of these devices and briefly discusses the benefits from the use of each.

SLANT BOARD

Slant boards can be purchased from sporting goods stores. They can also be made inexpensively. Cover a plank with some sort of padding, tack it down, and voila: you have a slant board. The board should be a little longer than you are tall and at least as wide as is your body with your arms by your side. Place the slant board at a 20-45° angle, then lie on it with your feet up and your head down. Rest in this position once or twice a day for fifteen to twenty minutes. The regular use of a slant board will improve your general circulation, relieve eyestrain and fatigue, improve hearing and vision, help sinus conditions, encourage new hair-growth, benefit your complexion, relieve the almost constant downward pull of gravity on your internal organs, improve the circulation in your legs and feet, and better your overall health. To relieve lower back strain, place a bolster cushion or two bed pillows under your knees and rest your head on a folded towel or small pillow that is approximately 1 1/2-2 inches thick.

FOOTSIE ROLLER

Footsie rollers can be purchased in your local health food store. With the purchase comes a brochure explaining how to use it. Regular use of your roller will improve the circulation to your legs and feet, as well as the flexibility of your knee joints. It will also improve your overall health, because the roller stimulates all the reflex points on the bottom of your feet which correspond to all your internal organs and all parts of your body. Use the footsie roller while reading, relaxing or watching television.

KENKOH SANDALS

These sandals have tiny, raised projections on the top surface of the sole of the shoe which constantly make contact with the sole of your foot. Walking with these sandals constantly stimulates all the reflex points on the soles of your feet, improves your overall circulation, and relieves tired, cold or aching feet. Wear the sandals only briefly at first, in order to allow your feet time to adjust to the constant stimulation.

TRAMPOLINE

Trampolining is fast becoming a very popular form of exercise. It's fun, and it really does do wonders to improve your overall health. Trampolining also burns more calories than most other types of exercise. So, if weight's your problem, this is the solution you've been looking for. Do not purchase one of the cheapest models, as it will not endure as much wear-and-tear as one better made. When beginning your exercise routine on the trampoline, position the trampoline near a wall so that you can use the wall for balance. Don't overdo it at first. Begin with one or two minutes at a time, then gradually increase the length of time you spend rebounding. The first time most people get on a rebounder, they are so excited that they jog and jump for five or ten minutes. The next day they regret it because their legs ache. It's not advisable to strain your muscles. Restrain your enthusiasm at the outset, and gradually lengthen the time you spend on your trampoline.

IONIZER

If you live in or near a large city, it is impossible to breathe clean air. Even country dwellers are now experiencing the results of polluted atmospheres. Your lungs, skin and liver could use a break. A top-quality ionizer will greatly improve the quality of the air you breathe. Two to four per room is ideal. Ionizers also improve your concentration and give you more energy.

HUMIDIFIER

The winter months leave your house much too dry for healthful living. A humidifier replaces the moisture needed to keep your skin young and healthy-looking. It also helps to improve your overall health. Purchase a top quality unit, otherwise you are wasting your money.

PLANTS

Fill your apartment or house with plants. They consume your carbon dioxide and produce fresh oxygen for you to breathe. Apart from this life-giving quality, they are beautiful to behold and sensitive, responsive friends to have in your home.

INVERSION BOOTS

Inversion boots are sold in sporting goods stores. You clip the boots onto your ankles and hook the boots onto a chin-up bar. Then you hang upside down. You can also do sit-ups or kneebends while hanging. Even if you do nothing but hang, you will improve your circulation, relieve eyestrain, encourage hair-growth, relieve sinus congestion, release low back pain and improve your complexion. Your general health will also improve. Be sure the chin-up bar is secure. Raise and lower yourself slowly, and you'll have no problems.

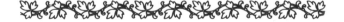

Organisations Of Interest To Readers Of This Book

It is still difficult to find many holistic doctors in the UK, though their numbers are increasing as more see the inherent restrictions of allopathic medicine and look for answers to their patients' problems elsewhere. Probably the best thing to do is to write to or telephone The Institute for Complementary Medicine, 21 Portland Place, London W1N 3AF (Tel. 01-636-9543), which will be able to give you the latest information about holistic doctors in your area.

The following pages list organisations in the UK that could be useful for the reader who wants to take a further interest in many of the subject areas mentioned in the book.

First, a list of addresses in the US for special products or services that are unavailable in the UK.

FOOD COMBINING

Simple Food Combining Wall Chart
Box 1858
Boulder, Colorado 80306
Services: Mail-order chart
The chart summarises a complicated subject very effectively in an easy-to-understand and attractive format.

FOOTSIE ROLLER

Matrix International
244 Brighton Avenue
Boston, Massachusetts 02134
Services: Manufacturer of footsie rollers. Most health food stores carry footsie rollers, but if you are unable to obtain one in your area, try writing to the above address.

INVERSION BOOTS

Gravity Guidance, Inc.
One West California Blvd.
Pasadena, California
Services: Mail-order inversion boots, Gravity Guider and Dr Robert Martin's book THE GRAVITY GUIDING SYSTEM

KENKOH SANDALS

Yaohan U.S.A. Corporation
431 Boyd Street
Los Angeles, California 90013
(213) 680-9001
Services: Mail-order sandals
Many health food stores also sell these wonderful sandals. Wear them after your shower or wear them all day. They massage your feet for you.

MUSIC

Steven Halpern Sounds
620 Taylor Way #14,
Belmont, California 94002
Services: Mail-order tapes and records of music appropriate for massaging, meditating or listening.

SWEDISH MASSAGE

Swedish Institute, Inc.
875 Avenue of the Americas
New York, New York 10001
(212) 695-3964
Services: Instruction, certification, preparation for licensing, massage practitioner references, graduate courses.

The Swedish Institute is the oldest massage school in the USA and the only massage school that is accredited by the US Department of Education.

OSTEOPATHY

British Naturopathic and
Osteopathic Association
6 Netherhall Gardens
London NW3 5RR
01 435 8728/7830

British College of Naturopathy &
Osteopathy
6 Netherhall Gardens
London NW3 5RR
01 435 7830

British & European Osteopathic
Association
General Secretary & Registrar
42/45 Broad Street
London EC2M 1QY
0233 31530

Andrew Still College of Osteopathy
94 Banstead Road
Sutton Surrey
01 642 4161
OR
53 Ross Road
London SE25
01 771 2014

Faculty of Osteopathy
21 St Albans Road
Lytham St Annes
Lancs FY8 1TG

European School of Osteopathy
(Osteopathic Education & Research
Ltd)
104 Tonbridge Road
Maidstone, Kent ME16 8SL

British School of Osteopathy
1-4 Suffolk Street
London SW1
01 930 9254

British Osteopathic Association
8-10 Boston Place
London NW1 6QH
01 262 5250

Osteopathic Medical Association
6 Dorset Street
London W1
01 580 6147

The General Council & Register of
Osteopaths
1 Suffolk Street
London SW1Y 4HG
01 839 2060

T'AI CHI CHUAN

School of T'ai Chi Chuan
49 The Avenue
London NW6
01 459 0764

London School of T'ai Chi Chuan
and Traditional Health Resources
PO Box 363
London NW2 6AF
01 586 7657

International T'ai Chi Chuan
Association
40 Hillcroft Gardens
Wembley Park
Middlesex
01 902 2351

British T'ai Chi Chuan Association
& London T'ai Chi Academy
7 Upper Wimpole Street
London W1
01 935 8444

TOUCH FOR HEALTH

Touch for Health Foundation
42 Worthington Road
Surbiton, Surrey KT6 7RX
01 399 7377

ROLFING

Nature Cure Clinic
15 Oldbury Place
London W1M 3AL
01 935 2787/6213

Rolf Institute
69 Marlborough Place
London NW8
01 624 3835

SHIATSU

Shiatsu Society
Secretary—Elaine Leichti
1 Railway Cottage
Thames Avenue
Pangbourne, Berks RG8 7BX

REFLEXOLOGY

Reflexology Centre
18 Deepdene Drive
Dorking, Surrey
01 464 9401 or Dorking 884254

Churchill Centre
22 Montagu Street
London W1H 1TB
01 402 9475

International Institute of
Reflexology
PO Box 34, 92 Sheering Road
Harlow, Essex CM17 OLT
Harlow 29060

Chiltern Institute of Reflexology
193 Tring Road
Aylesbury, Berks HP20 1JH

British School for Reflex Zone
Therapy of the Feet
Secretary—Ann Lett
151 Lichfield Grove
Finchley, London N3 2SL
01 629 3481

Bayley School of Reflexology
Monks Orchard
Whitbourne, Worcs
0886 21207

MASSAGE

West London School of
Therapeutic Massage
41 St Luke's Road
London W11 1DD
01 229 7411/4672

Northern Institute of
Massage/Northern College of
Physical Therapies
100 Waterloo Road
Blackpool, Lancs FY4 1AW
0253 403548

Natural Therapeutic Research Trust
3 Clement Gardens
Diss, Norfolk

Fylde School of Natural Therapies
21 St Albans Road
Lytham St Annes
Lancs FY8 1TG

Massage Tuition
David Mayer
2 Hall Cottages
Kingston Hall Farm
Nr Hitchin, Herts SG4 8EJ
0438 832994

International Federation of Manual
Medicine
28 Wimpole Street
London W1M 7AD
01 580 0391

HOMOEOPATHY

Society of Homoeopaths
101 Sebastian Avenue
Shenfield
Brentwood, Essex CM15 8PP
0227 224577

Faculty of Homoeopathy
Great Ormond Street
London WC1N 3HR
01 837 3091 Ex.72

College of Homoeopathy
7a Gilmore Road
Lewisham London SE13
01 852 0573

The British Homoeopathic
Association
Basildon Court
27a Devonshire Street
London W1N 1RJ
01 935 2163

British Association of
Homoeopathic Pharmacists
19a Cavendish Square
London W1M 9AD
01 629 3205

CHIROPRACTIC

Chiropractic Medical Association
51 Canford Cliffs Road
Poole, Dorset

British Chiropractors' Association
5 First Avenue
Chelmsford, Essex CM1 1RX
0245 353078
Executive Secretary:
69 Walton Park,
Pannel, Nr. Harrogate
N. Yorks HG3 1RJ
0423 870945

ALEXANDER TECHNIQUE

School of Alexander Studies
44 Park Avenue North
London N8
01 348 5054

Alexander Teaching Associates
ATA Centre
188 Old Street
London EC1V 9BP
01 250 3038

Alexander Technique Teachers'
Training Course
1 John's Avenue
London NW4
01 203 2851

ACUPUNCTURE

Register of British Acupuncturists
94 Banstead Road South
Sutton, Surrey SM2 5LH

Medical Acupuncture Society
15 Devonshire Place
London W1N 1PB
01 935 7575

International College of Oriental
Medicine
Green Hedges House
Green Hedges Avenue
East Grinstead
Sussex RH19 1DZ
0342 28567

British Medical Acupuncture
Society
Secretary—5 Sunningfields Road
London NW4

The British College of Acupuncture
Registrar Olga Orr
44 New Market Square
Basingstoke, Hants
Basingstoke 65333

British Association for Traditional
Chinese Medicine
c/o Lin Academy of Traditional
Chinese Medicine
13 Gunnersbury Avenue
Ealing Common
London W5 3XD
01 993 2549/992 2611

British Acupuncture Association &
Register
34 Alderney Street
London SW1V 4EU
OR
538 Forest Road
London E17 4NB
01 834 1012

Association of Western
Acupuncture
2 Rodney Street
Liverpool L1 2TE
051 709 0479

Acupuncture Research Society
34 Alderney Street
London SW1V 4EU
01 834 3353

IONISERS

Medion Ltd.
Beadles Lane
Oxted, Surrey

Index